How to Buy Wine at the Grocery Store

CARL W. DAVIS

How to Buy Wine at the Grocery Store

ISBN: 979-8-218-84025-9

Published by Blunderbuss Books

PO BOX 57281 New Orleans, LA 70112

The author expresses special thanks to Salem Roach for the inspiration to write this book and to Kristin Ramsey for her editorial guidance.

Table of Contents

Foreword

Wine has been part of human culture from time immemorial. One of the oldest Hebrew prayers is one that thanks God for wine. "Baruch atah, Adonai Eloheinu, Melech haolam, borei p'ri hagafen," translated to English as "Blessed Are You Adonai our God, King of the Universe, who has created the fruit of the vine!" Today, thousands of years after the first person said that prayer, we humans are still drinking wine and, especially when it is good wine, thanking God for it. Today, most literature about wine assumes that the reader has access to a vast wine store where every imaginable wine ever made is available, with every obscure varietal sitting on a shelf waiting to be procured. The reality is that most of us in America are getting our wine from a grocery store, with limited options available. We want to know what to buy from the options in front of us and within our budget. We want to know what to buy when we stop by a friend's house for dinner and don't want to arrive empty-handed. We want to know which bottle we should serve with dinner on Tuesday evening, and which one would go better with the food we are serving on Thursday. This book is for us, people who are in that great tradition of human history, enjoying wine, and getting it at the grocery store.

CHAPTER 1

In the Grocery Store

We have all been there. Standing in the wine aisle at the grocery store and wondering what to buy. We try to remember which wines we have had before that we liked, and which food we served them with that seemed to complement each wine. We are at the restaurant that we liked last month. We try to remember the name of a wine that a friend mentioned. We look at the cool pictures on the bottles and at the price tags. Then we grab something and hope we made a good selection.

Here are a few hints to make that process a bit more fun and productive. First, not all wines are created equal. Some are fine for drinking on their own, and others are best paired with food. There are some that will go with certain types of foods better than with others. Some wine types are intrinsically cheaper to produce than others. Also, there are some places in the world that make good wines at lower price points than would be expected, due to the economic situation in the country where the wine is made. Wines in these categories create the golden zone for grocery store wine shopping.

For instance, it costs a lot of money to make a very good Pinot Noir, so you aren't likely to find many, or any, of those in the average grocery store. However, there are very high-quality malbecs made at low price points. This is simply due to how hard or easy it is to grow the different grape varieties and the places in the world where those grape varieties are able to reach their maximum potential. You can have a bottle of high-quality malbec from Argentina, where that grape reaches its full potential, for

$20 or less. That is much less than a moderate quality pinot noir from France, where that grape reaches its fullest potential. This is because the malbec grape is easier to grow than the pinot noir grape, and the economic conditions in Argentina make their wine cheaper to Americans than wine from France. This means that at the grocery store, selecting a Malbec can get you a top-quality wine, but selecting a pinot noir may result in having a lower quality bottle with your dinner, even if the pinot noir costs more than the malbec. If you were to compare the highest quality pinot noir to the highest quality malbec, you may find you prefer the pinot. But you likely wouldn't prefer the pinot vs. malbec when you are limited to what is at the grocery store and what is at the $20 price point! Buying good wine at the grocery store is possible if we focus on the grape types that can produce high-quality wines at lower price points, and buy wines from places where economic realities allow the American dollar to go far.

One of the struggles of living in the United States is that most of the wine on the shelves comes from the United States. Why is this a problem? For that matter, why do so many lovers of wine focus on wines that aren't from the USA? The reason is pretty simple. In the United States, there are no regulations around wine labeling. This means it is very hard to know what you are getting when you buy an American wine. Other parts of the world regulate these things, and those regulations allow us to know what to expect when we read the label on a bottle. For instance, if a wine label says that it is a red wine from Burgundy, France, we know that it has to have been made with the pinot noir grape. We know how pinot noir grapes made in that area should taste, smell, and look. That allows us to know if it is the wine we want to pair with specific food or enjoy in a specific time and place. In short, we know exactly what we are getting. However, if we see a wine that says it is a red wine from California, then all we know is that the wine is red and it is from California. It could be sweet or dry. It could taste like anything. It could be made from any variety or blend of varieties. No rules govern it. Buying it is a 100% gamble. The only way to know what it is like is to buy it and taste it. If I am shopping for wine to go with the veal that I am making for supper, I don't want to take that gamble. I want to buy the known commodity. So, I buy a non-USA wine because those labels mean something due to regulations that exist outside of the USA. Of course, some American wines do voluntarily choose to give us some good information on their labels. It is helpful when they choose to disclose the variety of grapes used and the geographic region it is from. Knowing those things and the alcohol content that is on each label can help us make some generalizations about the wine, so our gamble is not 100% blind in those cases. If you love drinking American wines, I encourage you to do so and keep track of the details of the wines you try. Learn what the wines are like by trying them, and then you can draw upon your experiences and memory when buying them again. However, if you are standing in the grocery store aisle on your way to your friend's house for dinner, or want to make sure you get something that you know will go well with the salmon you have in your grocery cart, it is best to choose wines with labels that mean something.

WHAT TO BUY AND WHY

Food and Wine Pairings

What to drink with what you eat is probably the most important question to answer when selecting wine. When pairing wine with a meal, it is important to remember that food impacts wine more than wine impacts food. So, when choosing a wine and food combination, focus more on what impact the food will have on the wine than the impact of the wine on the food. It is easy for a delicate wine to be overpowered by a strong meal. Here are some general ideas to consider when pairing wine with food.

First, it is helpful to know a handful of traditional wine pairings. These traditional food and wine pairings have been around for ages for a reason – they work well. Knowing them is the best first step in choosing a good wine for dinner.

FOOD	WINE	WHY
Steak	Cabernet Sauvignon, Malbec	High Tannin wine vs. fat and protein
Roast Chicken	Beaujolais, Pinot Noir	Soft tannins go well with lean foul
Salmon, Duck	Pinot Noir	Food and wine are of equal intensity
Stilton Cheese	Port	Salty cheese vs. sweet wine
Truffles	Barolo, Barbaresco, Pinot Noir	Earthy food and earthy wine
Pasta with Tomato	Sangiovese, Barolo	Acidity of wine cuts through acidic sauce
Pasta with white sauce	Pinot Grigio	Wine's acidity cuts through cream
Fried Chicken	Sparkling Wine	Acidity and effervescence cut through the dish's richness and fat, while the bubbles cleanse the palate between bites
Fish	Sauv. Blanc, Chenin Blanc	Acidity of wine stands up to richness of fish, minerality can stand up to brine

Using the table above is a solid starting point that won't lead you astray. But of greater help is to learn some basic wine/food pairing principles.

1. **Match intensity.** If the food is full of strong flavors, serve a bold wine. If the food is delicate, serve a delicate wine. If the food is of medium intensity, serve a medium wine. Many people believe this is the single most important rule for pairing wine and food.

2. **Consider Acidity.** The general rule for food and wine pairing is that the wine should have a higher acidity than the food it's paired with. This is because food, particularly fatty, rich, or acidic dishes, can cause wine to taste flat or lifeless if the wine has lower acidity, whereas a higher-acidity wine acts to cleanse the palate, cut through fat, and enhance the overall flavors of the dish. High-acid white grapes include riesling, sauvignon blanc, and chenin blanc. A chardonnay from a cooler climate like Chablis will also be high in acidity. High-acid red grapes include cool-climate pinot noir, sangiovese, gamay, nebbiolo, and barbera.
3. **Consider Sweetness**. Your wine should always be as sweet or sweeter than the food you are eating. If your food is sweeter than your wine, it will make the wine taste sour and tart. For instance, this makes Rieslings a good match with things like sushi since both can be on the sweet side. The worst and most common food/wine pairing mistake is to serve a dry champagne with a sweet wedding cake. YUCK!

Sweet wine also pairs well with spicy dishes, salty foods, rich and creamy desserts, and fruit-based desserts. The key is to either complement the wine's flavors with similar notes or contrast the sweetness with contrasting tastes like salt, spice, or tartness. For sweet BBQ sauce, pair with a sweet white wine like Riesling or a sweeter red wine such as Zinfandel or Moscato, to complement the sauce's sweetness. Sparkling rosé is a versatile option that works well with various BBQ styles, including sweeter sauces, due to its fruitiness and refreshing acidity. Remember, you can usually tell a wine's sweetness level by looking at its Alcohol by Volume (ABV), which is printed on the label. Knowing this can help you select a wine with the desired dry/sweet level, even if the wine label does not say "dry" or "sweet," etc.

ABV	Sweetness Level
12.5% or More	Dry
11% to 12.5%	Off Dry
8% to 11%	Semi Sweet
8% or Less	Sweet

Here are some other things to remember:

1. The fattier the food, the more tannins the wine should have. This is because the tannins create a drying effect in the mouth that goes well with the greasy effect the fatty food has on the palate. Some wines with high tannins include: Nebbiolo, Cabernet Sauvignon, Syrah/Shiraz, Tempranillo, Sangiovese, Petite Sirah, and some Malbec (especially French).
2. Spicy Food makes the alcohol in wine seem harsh. So, serve sweeter wines as sweeter wines have lower alcohol than dry wines. The spice can also be softened by the sweetness of the wine. Many old Cajuns served sweet Sauterne wine with their spicy foods for this reason. Remember, when buying wine, look at the ABV on the label. The lower the ABV, the sweeter the wine.
3. Salt in food makes a wine taste less acidic, sweeter, and less bitter than it is. So, serve wines that are dry and have high acidity with salty foods.
4. Pair food and wine by place of origin. This school of thought says to serve Italian wine with Italian food, French wines with French food, Spanish wine with Spanish food, etc. Devotees of this method like to say, "What grows together goes together." This works well as long as the geographic location in question produces both good wine and good food!
5. Remember to consider the entire meal when pairing the wine. It is tempting to think only of the protein of the meal when deciding which wine to drink. But the entire meal must be considered.

Think especially about sauces. For instance, when thinking of what wine to pair with a "chicken dinner," it is very important to know if the chicken will be served with a tomato sauce, a mushroom sauce, or a lemon/butter sauce!

Let us put all of those guidelines into practice for buying wine at the grocery store to go with the meals we are going to eat at home this week. Our ideal list can't be followed 100% because we are limited to the good wines to be found in the average grocery store. If we had better access to wines, the list would be more robust. But considering what we have to work with, here we go!

MEAL	WINE
Spaghetti, Pizza, Ziti, Tomato Pasta	Chianti (ideally riserva or classico)
BBQ Ribs or BBQ chicken, BBQ Pork	Malbec (Ideally Mendoza), Sparkling Rosé
Meatloaf, Hamburgers, Ground Beef	Malbec (Ideally Mendoza)
Grilled Chicken	Pinot Grigio or Pinot Noir if it is from the Russian River Valley or Oregon
Salmon	Sauv blanc from New Zealand, or pinot noir from the Russian River Valley or Oregon
Steaks	Malbec (Ideally Mendoza)
Fettuccine Alfredo (alfredo pasta)	Pinot Grigio (Ideally Italian)
Grilled Seafood	Sauv blanc (New Zealand)
Mac & Cheese	Riesling (off dry or dry if possible), Cava
Fried Chicken/ anything deep fried	Cava or brut sparkling wine, if Cava is not available, Pinot Grigio
Fish	Sauv blanc (New Zealand)
Pork Chops	Tempranillo or Pinot Grigio (Ideally Italian) or pinot noir
Taco	Tempranillo or riesling
Grilled Cheese	Pinot Grigio, sauv. Blanc, or pinot noir
BLT	Sauv. Blanc, pinot noir, or Pinot Grigio
Sandwich (Salami or strong meats)	Chianti (Ideally riserva or classico) or Tempranillo
Sandwich Cold Cuts	Pinot Grigio

THE CHART EXPLAINED

Some grocery stores have great wine selections. Most have modest ones. If you don't know wine, it can be hard to tell the difference. Most grocery stores offer wine in the modest price category. In that category, you can find some very good wines if they come from a place where economic realities make wine cheap or if they are a type of wine that is inherently inexpensive to produce. In this chart, I looked at which wines the average grocery store has based on my experience, and I picked the best of that average selection and paired it with popular meals. Here is an overview of the wines and why they were selected:

1. Chianti (Ideally Classico or Riserva)

   Chianti is an Italian red wine originating from the Chianti region in Tuscany, Italy, made from the sangiovese grape (blend must be at least 80% sangiovese), and characterized by high acidity, robust tannins, and flavors of cherry, herbs, and earthy notes. It pairs well with rich, savory, and tomato-based Italian dishes like pasta and pizza. Historically, bottles of this wine were squat and wrapped in a straw basket. Many such empty bottles found a new life as a candle holder once the wine was consumed. These days, very little wine is bottled that way, but some still is. By law, all Chianti must be aged 6 months before it is bottled. Chianti, which is made in the most historic winemaking parts of Tuscany, considered by most to be the best places to make the wine, is called Chianti Classico and must be aged 12 months. If you have a choice, buy the classico. Chianti Classico Reserva is a wine that is aged 24 months and then must spend an additional 3 years in the bottle before release. If you have the option to buy Classico Riserva at your store, do so, especially if you want to enjoy the wine on its own, where you can better appreciate the nuance that it offers.

All Chianti, but especially classico and riserva wines, are of high quality and very enjoyable. They are a great companion to meals. That they are available at reasonable prices in most grocery stores is a product of current Italian economic realities, and we Americans can enjoy the situation.

2. Malbec (Ideally from Mendoza in Argentina)

   Malbec is a grape of French origin and named for Monsieur Malbeck, a Hungarian peasant who spread the grape across France, possibly in the 18th century. Although its original name was Côt, the grape became widely known as malbec after being planted in Bordeaux and later exported to Argentina, where it achieved its greatest success. It is a full-bodied red wine known for its deep color and flavors of dark fruits like blackberry and plum, as well as red fruit flavors like raspberry and sometimes notes of cocoa, tobacco, and leather. Argentinian Malbec often ends with a smooth, rich finish. Originally from France, it's now primarily associated with Argentina, where it thrives in the dry, sunny climate of regions like Mendoza, producing a signature style of lush, fruit-forward wine with softer tannins compared to French Malbec. It is a versatile wine, pairing well with meats, hearty stews, and even rich desserts like bittersweet chocolate. In the glass, the wine is very dark but has a magenta rim. Because the wine is well balanced, it is often enjoyed without food as well. Due to how well malbec grows in Argentina and the economic situation of the country, very high-quality Argentinian malbecs line our grocery shelves at very approachable price points. If you find one from Mendoza, you will not go wrong, and you won't break the bank. Due to the economic realities of Argentina, the highest quality wine to be found in most grocery stores (and on the wine lists of most mid-range restaurants) is an Argentine malbec. Many people tell me that their favorite wine is malbec. This is often because it is the only high-quality wine they have had, as it is the only truly high-quality wine offered where they get their wine.

3. Pinot Grigio (Ideally Italian)

   Pinot Grigio is a white wine with less than medium body, medium acidity, and medium alcohol. This means it goes with lots of different types of food. The wine is never aged or oaked; it is best consumed young. This keeps costs down because it costs money to age wine. The same grape makes wine in France, where it is called Pinot Gris, but due to economic factors, the Italian wine is less expensive and therefore more likely to be in your grocery store. Because this wine is cheap to produce and is so versatile, it is a great wine to get at the grocery store to have with dinner when a white wine is called for. You can expect flavors of lemon, lime, green apple, minerality, and salinity. Many American winemakers make Pinot Grigios. If you find one you like, please enjoy it. I suggest getting wines from Italy whenever possible because the standards they are required to meet ensure quality. American winemakers, having no standards to meet, often produce inferior products, and there is no way to know if the American wine you are buying is one of the good ones or not, other than trying it yourself. If you feel like gambling, try an American offering. Keep notes and buy the ones you like again. If you want to get a quality wine for sure, get Italian. High-quality versions of this wine can be found in grocery stores and at a lower cost because the grape is relatively inexpensive to grow, and the winemaking process does not require expensive aging. Therefore, this wine will always have a lower production cost than other wines, so high-quality examples can be had at a lower cost.

4. Pinot Noir (Russian River Valley or Oregon)

   Pinot noir grapes make some of the best wine on Earth. It is also one of the most expensive. Most associated with Burgundy, France, pinot noir is grown around the globe. This is a very difficult varietal for many reasons. One reason is that it is delicate and very hard to work with. It is easy to have a crop failure with this varietal. Next, it is extremely sensitive to its environment (called terroir). Wine made from these grapes will be drastically different simply because the grapes were grown feet apart. Because Burgundy makes exquisite wines from pinot noir, other places around the world have been trying to do the same for generations. They have not been successful. Most pinot noirs that are not from Burgundy disappoint greatly. However, in Oregon and in the Russian River Valley of Sonoma, California, some very good wines are made from the pnto noir grape. These examples are likely to be the only possibility of finding a good Pinot Noir wine in the average grocery store. The American wines will be heavier and more fruit-forward than wines from Burgundy, but still very good wines in their own right and likely to be among the most expensive wines on the shelf of the local grocery store. If you can find a Russian River Valley pinot noir in your grocery store, you will likely enjoy it! Good offerings from the Willamette Valley in Oregon may also be found in many grocery stores.

5. Sauvignon Blanc (New Zealand)

   Sauvignon blanc is one of the most popular grape varietals in the world. In France, wines made with this grape in Sancerre fetch top dollar and are highly prized. You are not likely to find a Sancerre or a Pouilly-Fumé at the grocery store for these reasons. However, the same grape grown in New Zealand is very affordable and delightful. Unlike the French wines that are more subtle, elegant, and mineral-driven, showcasing notes of citrus, white flowers, and flint, New Zealand Sauvignon Blanc is known for being aromatic, full-bodied, and bursting with tropical fruits like passionfruit, with a zesty, pungent character. It is by far the best value white wine in the grocery store. Marlborough is the part of New Zealand where excellent wines of this variety are made. You will not go wrong with a Marlborough Sauvignon Blanc from your grocery store. The economic realities of wine production in New Zealand, combined with the fact that this wine is made to be consumed while young and therefore does not require expensive aging, result in high-quality, low cost examples of New Zealand Sauvignon Blanc found at almost every grocery store in America.

6. Riesling

   Riesling is a white grape variety that originated in the Rhine area of Germany. It has historically been known as a sweet wine served in a slender blue bottle. Riesling is an aromatic grape variety displaying flowery, almost perfumed, aromas and has high acidity. Today, it is used to make dry, off-dry, semi-sweet, and sweet wines. Riesling is used to make both still and sparkling wines. Riesling wines are usually varietally pure and are seldom oaked. While historically sweet, today there is more dry Riesling being made than sweet Riesling. Look for Dry, Off Dry, or Semi-Sweet on the label when shopping for this wine to go with meals. If buying German Riesling, look for the words "Trocken," which means dry, or "Halbtrocken," which means semi-dry. Some good dry Rieslings are being made in Washington State that you are likely to find on your grocery store shelf as well.

7. Cava

   Many Americans are in the terrible habit of calling all sparkling wine Champagne. This is as silly as calling every automobile a Ford. Cava is a sparkling wine made in Spain using the same method that the French use to make Champagne. It is traditionally made from three white grape varietals: macabeo, xarel-lo, and parellada. Other authorized grapes include chardonnay, pinot noir, garnacha, monastrell, and trepat (for rosé Cava). Whereas Champagne is made from chardonnay, pinot noir, and pinot meunier. While made from different grape varietals, the method of making the wine is the same, giving Cava the same bread dough taste and feeling on the palate that Champagne gives, but at a fraction of the price due to the economic differences between Spain and France and the high profile that Champagne enjoys globally. You aren't likely to find a good Champagne at your grocery store, but you very well might find a good Cava. Be sure to serve the wine very cold.

8. Tempranillo

   You may see this wine sold under the name Rioja because wine from Rioja, Spain, is made from the tempranillo grape. This wine is known for its medium- to full-bodied, complex flavor profile, with notes of red fruit, spice, and leather, often complemented by vanilla and tobacco from oak aging. Tempranillo means "little early one," a name given due to the fact that it ripens early in the season. Due to the economic realities of Spain, this wine finds its way into our grocery stores at low prices and is very enjoyable alone or with food.

Bonus Good Finds in Grocery Stores:

1. Old Vine Zinfandel. The red grape we call zinfandel comes to us from Italy, where it is called primitivo and is grown in the Puglia region. DNA analysis has taught us that the wine came to Italy from what is now Croatia. During the time of Ancient Greece, the Greeks made much wine in the area that is now Croatia, and

it appears the Romans took this wine from the Ancient Greeks and began to grow it in Italy. Now we have it in California, too. In fact, this grape was one of the first wine grapes to be grown in California. This wine is one of the most ancient wines and is remarkably affordable. The Lodi area of California is the part of America where the climate is most like the growing climate in Italy, where the wine is grown. So, to have an American Zinfandel that is as close to an Italian Primitivo as possible, look for wines from Lodi, California. You will likely find them in your grocery store. Even though Lodi wine will be as close to the Old-World wine as is possible to make here, the American variety will be fruitier and jammier, and the Italian wine will be more earthy. The wine will have deep color, bold fruit-forward flavors like blackberry and plum, and often spicy notes of black pepper or licorice. It typically has medium-to-high acidity, moderate tannins, and high alcohol content (around 14-17% ABV), giving it a full-bodied and juicy texture. Treat yourself to one of the world's oldest wines at your grocery store.

2. Petite Sirah. Not to be confused with Sirah (also called Shiraz), Petite Sirah is a big-bodied red wine with high tannins and is a great companion to a steak dinner. It is also enjoyable on its own for those who like Big Reds. The wine is originally from France, and today, it is grown there as well as in Australia and the USA. Good examples of this wine can be found in grocery stores from time to time.

DON'T SHOW UP EMPTY-HANDED

If you are in the grocery store because you need to bring a bottle of wine to a friend's house and you don't know what to bring, look for a Malbec from Mendoza or a Russian River Valley Pinot Noir. If you prefer to bring a white wine, get a Sauvignon Blanc from New Zealand. If you wish to bring a sparkling wine, find a Cava.

A WORD ABOUT POINTS

In the 1980s, Robert Parker decided to develop a way to inform consumers about wine. At that time, very few wine writers were writing directly to the consumer. Most wrote only for other wine professionals. To help consumers find quality wines, he developed a 100-point wine rating system. However, the drinkable portion of that scale starts at 80. So, it is really a 20-point scale. Today, many different wine critics use point systems to grade wines. The point system can be summed up as follows:

- **Less than 80:** Wines are flawed.
- **80-84** wines are 'good'
- **85-90** wines are 'good' to 'very good'
- **90-94** wines are 'superior' to 'exceptional'
- **95-100** wines are benchmark examples or 'classic'

If you shop in a grocery store that has wines that have been awarded points, this can be a helpful way to know the quality to expect from the bottle. You still need to decide if that type of wine is what you will enjoy drinking or matches well with the meal you are preparing.

CHAPTER 2

What Makes a Wine "Good"

People often say some wines are "good" and others aren't, and it is assumed that means the person likes the wine or doesn't like the wine. Of course, if you like the wine you are drinking, then it is "good for *you,*" and that is ultimately what matters, since wine is meant to be enjoyed by the drinker! But that is not what we are talking about here. When we say a "wine is a good wine," we aren't saying it is a wine we like. We are saying it is a wine that meets certain quality standards. Here are some agreed-upon standards that don't have to do with individual preferences but that define a well-made, or "good" wine.

First, good wines are balanced. This means that their traits are in proportion to each other. Here are four major traits that all wines have: 1. Acidity 2. Alcohol level 3. Sweetness level 4. Tannin level. For a wine to be considered well-balanced, all these parts must exist in the proper ratio to each other. Each of these components plays a vital role in the creation of a good bottle of wine; too much of one part and the wine will suffer, not enough of a specific component and the wine will be lacking. For instance, the acid in the wine balances out the sweetness from the sugar, creating crisp, zingy flavor profiles. If there is too much acidity, the wine will cause your lips to pucker unpleasantly. But if there is not enough acidity, your wine will feel flat and flabby. Therefore, for a wine that is sweet to be well balanced, it must have correspondingly high acidity. A balanced wine has good structure. The term structure refers to the balance of a wine's core components: alcohol, acidity, tannins, and sweetness, which together create its overall body and mouthfeel. A well-structured wine is harmonious, with no single element overpowering the others, resulting in a balanced wine.

Next, consider the intensity of the wine. Intensity refers to the concentration of a wine's color, aroma, and flavor. Intensity is a measure of how pronounced or potent these characteristics are, with common descriptors, including pale, medium, and deep for color, light, medium, and pronounced for aroma and flavor. A higher intensity indicates a more concentrated and flavorful wine, while lower intensity suggests a milder, gentler, more delicate wine.

Next, consider length of finish. This refers to how long you continue to taste pleasant flavors after you have swallowed the wine. A longer, more persistent finish indicates higher quality, with desirable qualities continuing to be perceived for a significant duration of time, sometimes even a minute or more, whereas a short finish fades quickly.

Finally, consider complexity. Does the wine offer many sensory experiences? Does it have more than one flavor and more than one aroma? Or is it all just one smell and one flavor? Wines that do more than one thing at once are more complex, and wines that do not are considered simple.

Evaluate the wine you are drinking based on the above criteria. A wine scoring high in each of the above four aspects is generally considered outstanding or very good, while a wine with only one or two of these characteristics might be considered average or poor. A good wine will have at least three of them. Remember, just because you don't like a wine doesn't mean it is automatically "bad" - one person's trash is another's treasure. Using these metrics to judge wine helps us get away from calling something good or bad just because we do or do not like it, and instead sets independent quality standards for what a "good wine" truly is. When we say a wine is "good," we mean it is of good quality, though we may or may not like it personally.

CHAPTER 3

How to Drink Wine

Believe it or not, there is a process to drinking wine that is designed to provide the most pleasure possible from the experience!

The first step in enjoying wine is removing it from the bottle. To open a bottle of still wine (not sparkling) that is closed with a cork, first remove the top part of the capsule. The capsule is the foil covering over the cork. Most cork screws have a small, curved knife built into them for this purpose. In olden times, this foil was made of lead, and so removing it was essential to keep the wine from contacting the toxic material. Today, different metals are used, but the need to remove the metal from the mouth of the bottle remains. After the capsule has been removed, wipe the neck of the bottle with a cloth to ensure no tiny bits of foil can get into the wine when the cork is removed. Center the corkscrew in the middle of the cork and screw it into the cork, and then pull the cork out gently. Many corkscrews have fold-down prongs to catch the neck of the bottle, allowing the cork to be removed with the help of leverage. Once the cork is removed, wipe the bottle's mouth with a clean cloth. To open a bottle of sparkling wine, a different technique is used. First, make sure the wine is well chilled. There is much pressure in the bottle, and chilling helps to ensure the wine does not come exploding out when the stopper is removed. Next, remove the foil that covers the wire cage. Then carefully loosen, but do not remove the wire cage. Do this by twisting the wire tie-down 6 times. The wire cage will stay on the bottle during the entire opening process. From the time the wire cage is loosened, keep your hand or thumb over the cork to prevent it from flying out, and always be sure the bottle is pointed in a safe direction. Then hold the bottle at an angle, pointed away from yourself and other people. Hold the cork firmly so that the pressure in the bottle doesn't force it out too fast. Then, holding the cork still, turn the bottle until the cork comes free.

WHEN YOU CAN AND CAN'T DECANT

Wines that have been aged in the bottle may benefit from decanting. Other wines may be ruined by decanting. Here are some general rules to decide if you should decant or not.

YES – Decant These Wines

A. Old Red Wines with Sediment:

Mature wines, typically 10 years or older, often develop sediment at the bottom of the bottle. Decanting separates the clear wine from the sediment, which can have a negative impact on flavor.

B. Young, Tannic Red Wines:

Wines with a strong, robust structure and high tannin levels can benefit from aeration. The oxygen in the decanter helps to soften the tannins and make the wine smoother and more approachable.

C. "Reduced" Wines:

Some wines, particularly natural wines, can exhibit a reduced or "closed" nose with unpleasant odors like burnt matches. Decanting can help to "burn off" these sulfurous compounds and allow the desired fruit and floral aromas to return. "Reduced" wines are further discussed in Chapter Nine of this book.

D. Rich White Wines:

Fuller-bodied white wines and some rosés can also benefit from decanting, especially if they are young and need to open up their flavor profiles and aromatics.

NO - DO NOT DECANT THESE WINES

A. Sparkling Wines:

Decanting will cause the wine to go flat by releasing the carbonation that gives it its characteristic bubbles.

Extremely Old / Fragile Wines:

While older wines are typically decanted for sediment, very delicate wines (e.g., 40-50 years or more) are too fragile for the aeration process.

B. Light Fruity Wine:

Lighter-colored, young wines that are already fruity and fragrant don't need decanting.

Related to decanting is the idea of letting the wine breathe. This means allowing the wine to be exposed to air. Decanting is one way to do that. However, wine can be allowed to breathe simply by waiting between when the bottle is opened and when the wine is poured into the glass. Wine can also be allowed to sit in the glass before being consumed, and it can be aerated by simply swirling it in the glass. Several gadgets on the market help wine breathe. They are usually pretty glass tubes through which the wine is poured. While these may work, they are not needed. The traditional methods of exposing wine to air work just fine. Generally, young fruity reds and almost all whites do not need to be decanted before being enjoyed. They may benefit from a swirl or two in the glass, but that is all that is needed. On the other hand, young wines with harsh tannins may benefit from being allowed to sit before being consumed for 30 minutes to 2 hours. Wines with noticeable sediment should be decanted.

Wine should be served in stemware. This allows for the best temperature control. By holding the wine glass by its stem, you do not transfer your body heat into the wine. If the wine is too cold and you want to warm it up, you can hold the glass by the bowl and do so with your body heat. Stemware gives you the most control and is therefore the best way to serve wine. Wine glasses are also designed so that the aroma of the wine will rise and collect at the mouth of the glass, allowing the drinker to enjoy the fragrance of the wine as much as possible. Also, the glass is designed to allow the drinker to view the wine as well as smell and taste it. Enjoying wine involves all of the senses. What about hearing, you ask? That is where the tradition of clinking glasses comes from. By clinking the glass with someone else who is enjoying wine, even the sense of hearing is added to the experience. For this process to work, the glass has to be properly filled. Too many people overfill the glass, and that prevents ideal smelling and viewing of the wine. If your wine glass has a wide middle and then narrows to the top, fill the wine glass only to its widest point in the bowl. If the glass does not have that tulip shape, only fill the bottom 1/3 of the glass.

The first step in enjoying the wine after it is poured into the glass is to view it. To do this, lift the glass into the light to see it well. Holding the glass by the stem, tilt the glass away from you about 45 degrees and look at the wine in the glass. The first thing to note is coloration. The next thing to note is clarity. Look to see if the wine changes color along the rim of the glass. Enjoy its visual beauty!

Next, smell the wine. Bring the glass under your nose and inhale. What does it smell like? Enjoy the fragrance!

Finally, bring the glass to your lips and taste it. Drink the wine and enjoy experiencing the expression of the time and place of that wine's creation.

COLORATION

Wine gets classified by color. We usually think of wine as being Red, White, or Rosé (Blush). However, within each of these broad categories, there is a spectrum of color from light to dark. The color of a wine can tell you much about the wine. The color is determined by things such as what grape varietal the wine is made from. Red wine made from grapes with dark, thick skins will be darker than red wines made from grapes with thinner or lighter skins. It can also tell you much about the winemaking process. For instance, a white wine that is not aged in oak will usually be much lighter in color than a white wine that is aged in oak.

Wine aficionados have developed standardized definitions of wine colors. To start with, it is helpful to consider just a few of those colors. White wine can range from almost clear like water to deep gold. Red wines can range from a dark pink to a deep purple. While wine experts will have many different labels for the variations on that spectrum, it can be helpful for the beginner to simply think of the following colors. For white wines: 1. Pale yellow (also called pale lemon) 2. Medium yellow (also called medium lemon) 3. Golden.

For red wines: 1. Ruby 2. Garnet.

To get an idea of these colors and compare them to each other, I suggest doing a tasting exercise with the following wines and observing their color in the glass:

Glass 1: Sauvignon Blanc from New Zealand (pale lemon)

Glass 2: Chardonnay from California (medium lemon)

Glass 3: Sauterne (gold)

Glass 4: Pinot Noir (medium ruby)

Glass 5: Malbec (garnet)

Generally speaking, the pale lemon wines will be younger, acidic (zesty), fresh, and often (but not always) from cooler climates. Wines in the medium lemon range may have been aged in oak, which will make a Chardonnay buttery and impart a complexity to the drinking experience. They often are fuller and more complex than pale wines. The golden wine in this example is a sweet dessert wine, and you will note the taste of honey-like sweetness. This is because the residual sugar in this wine is high and contributes to the darker color. A general rule is that a lighter wine may be drier, and a darker wine may be sweeter. But this is not always the case, just a rule of thumb. Wines in the medium ruby category are made from grapes with lighter skins and will, therefore, be less tannic than darker wines that are exposed to thicker, darker skins during the winemaking process, such as a Malbec. Also, as a wine ages, it may become more brown in color, so seeing a brownish tint to the wine may indicate the wine is older. Knowing these few things about color can help you quickly identify wine traits just from looking at it! This is why the first step in tasting wine is to view it in the glass.

After you view the wine, the next thing to do is to smell it. We are all familiar with the caricature sommelier who talks about exotic smells and imagery when nosing a wine. It is easy to dismiss this as pretense or artistic creativity. In many cases, there can be some of that. However, the fact is that there is a science behind why wine smells and tastes the way it does, and knowing a few basic facts about the chemistry of wine and how the chemical makeup of wine causes it to have specific aromas and flavors will go a long way to helping a person better understand and enjoy the wine they are consuming. Certain wine varieties are famous for having specific smells and flavors. Learning these can help you identify those varieties from their scent or "nose."

Here are some helpful hints for nosing and tasting wines. Some of these scents may not sound pleasant, but in the context of drinking the wine, they actually are. Learning to identify these common smells and flavors, knowing the chemical reason they are there, and in which wines you will find them, will do much to help you better enjoy the wines you find at the grocery store.

Here is a list of common wine aromas and flavors, the chemical reason for the aroma/flavor, and wine varietals that commonly exhibit these aromas/flavors:

RED FRUIT

(Raspberries, Strawberries, Red Cherries, Red Plum, Red Currants, etc.)

Chemical compounds in the wine, called esters, are produced during the fermentation process when yeast reacts with the acid. Different combinations of acids, along with fermentation temperature and yeast type, create esters that also appear in certain red fruits. These, therefore, contribute distinct "red fruit" aromas and flavors such as strawberry, raspberry, red plum, and cherry to wine.

As expected, red fruit aromas and flavors are found in red wines. Pinot Noir is known for cherry and raspberry notes, Gamay (Beaujolais), offering strawberry and cherry; Grenache, with flavors of red berries; and Merlot, which famously offers the aroma and flavor of plums.

BLACK FRUIT

(Blackberries, Black Cherry, Black Plum, Black Currant, etc.)

The black fruit taste in wine comes from several chemical compounds, primarily norisoprenoids and esters, which develop in the grape and evolve during fermentation and aging. Specific characteristics, such as black pepper or herbaceous notes, are contributed by other compounds like rotundone and methoxypyrazine.

Black fruit flavors and aromas are found in red wines such as Cabernet Sauvignon, Syrah/Shiraz, Malbec, Merlot, Zinfandel, Tempranillo, Petite Sirah, and, less commonly, in Pinot Noir.

CITRUS

(Lemon, Lime, Orange, Grapefruit, Tangerine)

Citrus can be perceived in some white wines and comes from a variety of naturally occurring chemical compounds, primarily terpenes and thiols, which are present in the grapes and are released during the winemaking process.

Some wines that are often identified with citrus are Chardonnays from colder climates, such as Chablis, as well as Riesling, Grüner Veltliner, and some Sauvignon Blanc.

APPLE/PEAR

Many white wines will have apple flavors that come from a combination of chemical compounds, primarily malic acid and certain esters, with specific characteristics influenced by winemaking techniques. Pear flavor in wine primarily comes from specific volatile chemical compounds produced during fermentation by yeast. The most significant pear-like esters are Ethyl Acetate and Isoamyl Acetate. Some wine varietals famous for these flavors and aromas are Pinot Grigio, Sauvignon Blanc, Veuve Clicquot, and Moscato.

STONE FRUIT

(Peaches, Nectarine, Apricot)

The primary chemical reasons for stone fruit flavors like peach and apricot in wine come from specific aromatic compounds, including lactones, terpenes, and specific esters. Wines famous for this are: Viognier, Roussanne, Marsanne, Riesling, Chenin Blanc, and Grenache Blanc, as well as some Chardonnays and Verdejo. Red wines like Sangiovese can also exhibit stone fruit characteristics.

TROPICAL FRUIT

(Pineapple, Mango, Passion Fruit, Papaya)

Tropical fruit flavors in wine are primarily caused by three groups of volatile compounds: thiols, esters, and terpenes. Famously, Sauvignon Blanc (especially from New Zealand), Chardonnay from warmer climates, Viognier, Chenin Blanc, Gewürztraminer, and Albariño offer notes of tropical fruit. The flavor profile of these wines is influenced by the concentration and interaction of these compounds. Additionally, some strains of yeast can cause tropical fruit flavor as well.

MELON

(Cantaloupe, Honeydew)

Like other aromas and flavors in wine, the perception of melon is caused by the chemical compounds called esters in the winemaking process. Wine varietals that can have melon flavor notes include Melon de Bourgogne (Muscadet), Gewürztraminer, Chardonnay, and Riesling. Other white wines like Pinot Grigio, Sauvignon Blanc, Albariño, and Vermentino can sometimes exhibit subtle melon nuances.

BEYOND THE FRUITY: BELL PEPPER

The phrase used to describe the smell of bell pepper in a wine is "vegetal aroma." The bell pepper flavor in certain wines is caused by methoxypyrazines, often simply called pyrazine. These organic chemical compounds are highly aromatic. The most significant methoxypyrazine responsible for the green bell pepper aroma is 3-isobutyl-2-methoxypyrazine, often referred to as IBMP.

These aromas and flavors are famously found in Bordeaux grape varieties, such as cabernet sauvignon, merlot, cabernet franc, as well as in carménère and sauvignon blanc. The intensity of this flavor depends on factors like climate, with cooler regions producing more pronounced green notes. While some consider it a flaw (especially in red wines), others enjoy this herbaceous characteristic, especially in white wines. It is a classic feature of New Zealand Sauvignon Blanc and of Chile's Carménère wine. It can also be part of a well-balanced Bordeaux blend.

FRESH CUT GRASS

Like the aroma of bell pepper, the aroma of grassiness in wine also comes from methoxypyrazines. Sauvignon Blanc is famous for being grassy.

EARTH

Some wines will smell and taste of the Earth, or dirt. Words people often use to describe this are forest floor, compost, mushroom, potting soil, or fresh turned soil. When a wine is described positively as having notes of forest floor, it is typically referring to savory, earthy aromas such as mushrooms, truffles, and damp earth. Geosmin is an organic compound that is responsible for the classic smell of soil and is produced by certain bacteria and fungi during the winemaking process. Additionally, in the vineyard, bacteria like Streptomyces often found in clay-rich or wet soils, can be taken up by grape skins and transferred to the wine. At low concentrations, geosmin can contribute to a desirable earthy character, even in young wines, especially in varieties like Pinot Noir. Some people famously call this "Pinot Noir Funk." Moreover, the sulfur compound Dimethyl Sulfide (DMS) can also contribute to notes of earthiness. DMS develops during bottle aging and is a sign of aged wines because, as a wine matures, its initial fruity aromas fade and complex tertiary aromas, like mushrooms, dried leaves, and tobacco, can emerge. This natural aging process allows the forest floor characteristics to evolve. So, earthy notes can be present in some young wines and also in aged wines, but for different reasons.

MINERAL

(Wet stone, limestone, chalk, slate, flint)

These notes, famously found in cool-climate chardonnay wines such as Chablis and in some Sauvignon Blancs, especially those from the Old

World, like Sancerre or Pouilly Fumé, come from trace levels of volatile sulfur compounds and other minerals in the soil where the grapes are grown. At low concentrations, these aromas are considered a desirable sign of complexity. At higher levels, they become a fault known as "reduction," characterized by unpleasant smells of rotten eggs or burnt rubber. Sulfur compounds are often produced by yeasts during fermentation, especially in musts with low nitrogen content or when excess elemental sulfur from vineyard treatments is present. Some winemakers even use techniques that encourage reductive characters to achieve a flinty style. As with many traits, in small amounts they are desirable and add to the wine's character, but in too large a dose, they become a fault. Generally speaking, Old World wines have more minerality than New World wines. Wine from the same grape varietal grown in the New World will tend to be more fruit-forward and full-bodied than their Old-World counterparts, which will often be less fruit-forward and have higher minerality.

FLOWERS

Floral notes come from chemical compounds called terpenes. Hints of geranium and rosé are caused by terpenoid geraniol. Linalool is a terpene that creates delicate notes of lily and orange blossom, while ketones and diketones will give lavender fragrance to a wine. The smell of elderflower and linden blossoms comes from the terpene hotrienol.

Some wines noted for having floral characteristics are Chenin Blanc, Albarino, Semillon, Gewrüztraminer, Riesling, Viognier, and even some reds like Nebbiolo, Cabernet Sauvignon, and Syrah, as well as Sangiovese.

WOOD/OAK

(Cedar, Leather, Vanilla, Smoke, Baking Spices such as Cinnamon, Clove & Nutmeg)

The taste and aroma of leather, oak, and cedar in wine are not from the grapes themselves but from specific chemical compounds that develop during the winemaking process and aging. These compounds are primarily extracted from oak barrels or produced by the metabolism of yeast. The leathery taste and aroma in wine can come from two distinct sources, one of which is generally considered a fault. The first option is aged tannins. As red wine ages, tannins — complex phenolic compounds from grape skins and seeds, and oak barrels — polymerize and form larger, smoother chains. This mellows the wine's astringency and can result in complex aromas described as leathery or savory. Secondly, it can be caused by Brettanomyces yeast. The presence of this "wild yeast" produces volatile phenols that give aromas reminiscent of leather, barnyard, and horse saddles. While high levels are considered a wine fault, some people appreciate the woodsy, leathery notes at lower concentrations.

HOW THEY GOT THERE

The aromas and flavors in the wine we drink enter the wine during one of three stages. First, we have primary aromas. These are inherent to the grape variety itself and can include fruity, herbal, and floral notes. Next, we have the aromas and flavors that came into the wine during the winemaking process. We call these secondary aromas. These aromas develop from the winemaking process, particularly during fermentation. Examples of secondary aromas in wine include vanilla, toast, and smoke from oak barrel aging, as well as buttery or creamy notes from malolactic fermentation and biscuity or yeasty notes from lees aging. These notes are produced during the winemaking (vinification) process, rather than coming directly from the grape itself, such as being a result of fermentation, oak exposure, and other post-fermentation techniques. Therefore, they are called secondary. Finally, there is Tertiary Aroma. These aromas come from bottle aging. Some wines can be stored for long periods of time in their bottles and are very enjoyable when finally consumed. These wines develop unique aromas and flavors during that time of bottle storage. These notes are said to be tertiary aromas and will vary greatly from bottle to bottle. Examples of tertiary aromas include notes of leather, earth, or dried fruit.

So as you can see, there is a science behind how wine smells, looks, and tastes! There are actually chemical compounds in the wine that cause it to smell like "fresh cut grass" or "the floor of damp woods." These descriptors are not "wine poetry" alone. Albeit some people (usually the less informed) will certainly go far down the path of creative writing when describing wine, sticking to the descriptors above, based solidly on the chemistry of the wine, is a solid way to understand, enjoy, and express the experience of wine. Appreciating wine involves science and art, but most of all, it is a joy!

The broad list of aromas and flavors above is a good starting place. They are simple but solid enough to help the wine enthusiast identify and enjoy their wine. They don't have to be an endpoint, however! People studying to work professionally in the wine industry will often buy smell kits that have small vials of different smells. They will spend hours smelling these vials and memorizing the names of each unique smell, thereby building their smelling vocabulary, so that they can identify as many subtleties in the wines they serve and enjoy as much as possible. They will also taste as many different flavors as possible and remember them so that they can better describe the flavors found in wine. But for most of us who buy our wine at the grocery store, the simple list above will put us on solid ground.

TASTING

In most cases, the taste of the wine will reflect the smell of the wine. For instance, if your wine smelled of fresh red fruits like strawberries and cherries, you would likely taste the flavor of strawberries and cherries when you drink the wine. The same chemical process that causes the wine to have the same scent as those fruits will cause it to have the same flavor too. However, sometimes a scent may be prominent on the nose but subtle on the palate, or the other way around. Paying attention to these variations is part of the process of enjoying wine. There are also many times when you will taste something you didn't smell, or smell something you didn't taste. This reality is different from person to person since everyone's sensitivity levels are different. One person may be more sensitive to smell than to taste or vice versa. Sometimes, after you taste a flavor, you will notice it the next time you smell the wine, even though you didn't smell it the first time. Sometimes the taste is not what was expected based upon the smell, and a surprise is enjoyed. It is a fun process! Wines that have one primary taste and flavor are said to be simple, whereas wines that have many tastes and flavors happening at the same time, or over the course of drinking the wine, are said to be complex. Wines that leave a pleasant flavor in your mouth for a noticeable period of time after swallowing are said to have a long finish. Often, the flavor the wine leaves will change over time before disappearing. These wines are said to have a complex finish. Wines that you can't taste long after you swallow are said to have a short finish. Logically, wines in between a medium finish. Take time between sips to experience the finish and notice if it changes.

How wine is served is of the utmost importance. Even the best wine cannot be fully enjoyed if it is not properly served. Fortunately, serving a wine well is not difficult. There are a few things to focus on. The first is temperature. We Americans have a hard time with this because, for years, we have been told things like "serve red wines at room temperature." The problem with that advice is that it comes to us from Northern Europe, where "room temperature" is around 65 degrees Fahrenheit. This advice does not work globally. I live in New Orleans, Louisiana, where a cool room is one that is 73 degrees. Generally speaking, we tend to drink our whites too cold and our reds too warm. If you store your white wine in the refrigerator, take it out about 30 minutes before opening the bottle. If you keep your red wines in a rack, put the bottle in the refrigerator about 30 minutes before opening the bottle. This will allow the wines to come to a better temperature for service. Another good rule of thumb is that lighter white wines should be served colder and heavier red wines warmer. Medium wines, such as a white wine that is a fully oaked Chardonnay or a red wine that is a delicate red Burgundy, should be served in the middle, neither too cold nor too warm. Here is a temperature chart by wine type for ideal wine service.

Wine	Service Temperature
Sparkling Wine	40-50 Degrees F
Ice Wine	45-50 Degrees F
Light White Wine	45-50 Degrees F
Heavy White (Oaked Chard, etc.)	45-50 Degrees F
Light Red (Red Burgundy, Beaujolais, etc.)	45-50 Degrees F
Tawny Port	57-60 Degrees F
Ruby and Vintage Port	60-65 Degrees F
Heavy Red Wine	60-68 Degrees F

To chill wine using an ice bucket, fill the bucket with half cold water and half ice, instead of filling it with ice alone. The cold water will have more surface contact with the bottle than ice alone does, thus cooling the wine more efficiently.

The next important thing to consider when serving wine is the glassware. Use stemmed glasses. Stemmed glasses serve an important function. They allow the drinker to control the temperature of the wine by how the glass is held. To keep the wine cool, the glass is held by the stem to limit the transfer of heat from the hand to the glass. To warm up the wine, the glass is held by the bowl to transfer heat. Stemware also allows the drinker to hold the wine glass by the stem and truly look at the wine without having the view obscured by fingers. Stemware keeps fingerprints off the bowl of the glass so that the wine can be better viewed in the light. Most importantly, the glasses must be clean! Sometimes, glasses can develop a bad smell from being washed with less-than-ideal dishwater or from being put away while wet, thus allowing odors to develop in the storage cabinet. Fix these problems before adding wine to the glass. Do not overfill the glass. A wine glass should be filled to its widest point if the bowl of the wine glass flares. This is usually just below the middle of the glass. If the bowl of the wine glass does not flare, then it should be filled 1/3 of the way full. This allows the wine to be moved in the glass by swirling to observe things such as the alcohol content by observing the legs or tears that form on the glass. These are clear liquids that stay on the side of the glass and drip down the glass after you swirl the wine to expose the wine to the sides of the glass. Wines with higher alcohol content form slower-moving tears on the sides of the glass than wines with lower alcohol contents do. A wine with a higher alcohol content, producing slower-dripping legs, will likely be dry. We can visually perceive these features when the glass is correctly filled. Filling to this level also allows the glass to be tilted so that the rim of the wine can be seen and the color, clarity, and intensity appreciated visually. Swirling the wine exposes it to air and allows different aromas and flavors to be noticed. There are different types of glasses for different types of wine. Red wine glasses have larger, wider bowls to maximize oxidation and release complex aromas, while white wine glasses have narrower bowls and smaller rims to preserve delicate aromas and maintain lower serving temperatures. Red wines are bolder and sometimes need more air to develop, whereas white wines are sometimes fragile, requiring a shape that concentrates their subtler floral and fruit notes. However, a general-purpose stemmed wine glass can be used for almost any wine with great adequacy. Separate red/ white glasses are not needed, but they are a nicety. Sparkling wine is traditionally served in a coupe or flute. However, many people prefer to enjoy it in a typical stemmed glass as well, especially sparkling wines made in the Traditional Method, as those wines have interesting flavors of bread from exposure to the yeast in the bottle during production, and many people find these flavors can be better appreciated in a traditional wine glass.

ORDERING WINE AT A RESTAURANT

When you order a bottle of wine at a restaurant, the wine will be served according to an established process. First, the waiter will bring the bottle of wine to the table and show it to the person who ordered it. The reason for this is so that you can confirm that the waiter has brought the correct wine. Review the label and make sure it is what you selected from the menu. Next, the waiter will open the wine. The cork will then be displayed to the person who ordered the wine and placed on a small coaster on the table. The reason for this is so that you can get an idea of whether the wine was stored correctly. Wine should be stored horizontally so that the wine is always in contact with the cork. This stops the cork from drying out and the wine from spoiling. You should expect to see evidence of wine contact on the bottom of the cork. If you don't, that can be a warning sign. The next thing the server will do is pour a small amount of wine into the glass of the person who ordered it. This is so you can check it for faults. Pick up the glass, hold it at an angle tilted away from you, and look at the wine. You are looking to make sure that nothing is floating in it and that it looks as you would expect it to look.

In the faults section of this book, visual clues to faults are discussed. You are looking for those. After that, you might swirl the wine in the glass. There is only a small amount of wine poured into your glass to make this easy. This creates air contact with the wine, which can enhance aroma and taste. Next, smell the wine. This is where most faults can be detected. If it smells like nail polish remover, rotten eggs, or moldy cardboard, the wine is flawed. After you have smelled the wine, you can finally drink the wine. Don't gulp it. Allow it to spend time in your mouth and move it around in your mouth to make contact with the different areas of your mouth where you taste different flavors. You are not drinking it to see if you like it. You are drinking it to make sure it is not flawed and exhibits the characteristics of the wine you selected. After you swallow, assuming the wine is not flawed, simply nod or tell the server, "Yes." The server will then serve the wine to the others at the table. The server will fill the glasses of the others at the table in a clockwise pattern, serving women first, then gentlemen, and finally the host, using a napkin in their left hand. The goal is to serve everyone an equal amount of wine, ensuring no one is singled out, and to keep the glasses consistently filled.

CHAPTER 4

How Wine is Made

Wine comes in three basic categories: Red, White, and In Between. This makes intuitive sense because some grape varieties have dark skins and some have light skins. The type of grape a wine is made from and how a wine is made determine which of these categories it fits into. It is logical to assume that dark grapes make red wine, and light grapes make white wine. However, as we will see, it is not quite that straightforward.

For instance, a white wine can be made from a red grape by keeping the skin of the grape out of the winemaking process. Conversely, a wine style that is currently popular, called "Orange Wine," that falls in the "in between red and white" category, is made by using white grapes and exposing the white grapes to the grape skins in the winemaking process. Traditionally, wine skins are only used in the process for red winemaking. Orange Wines are basically white wines made with light grapes using the process traditionally used for red wines. Clear as mud? The best way to understand the difference between these categories is to look, step by step, at how they are made. This is what makes a wine red, white, or in between.

Red and Rosé wines are made with dark grapes. Most commonly, people refer to these grapes as "black grapes," but some people will also call them "red" or simply "dark." This book will use these terms interchangeably. These dark grapes make red wine. Here are the steps taken when red or rosé wine is made.

1. Harvest the grapes. This can be done by hand or by machine. Regardless of the harvest method used, it must be done at exactly

the right time in the grape's development, so that the grape has the characteristics that the winemaker is seeking. For instance, wines made from grapes harvested early will have a different sugar content than wines made from grapes harvested late. The winemaker decides what he or she is seeking in the wine they are making and then harvests at the time of grape development, where the grapes offer the desired characteristic. The ripening of the grape is highly impacted by temperature, sun exposure, amount of moisture, the angle of the hill that the grape is planted on (aspect), and many other factors. The winemaker must take all of these factors (broadly referred to as the wine's terroir) into account when deciding when to harvest.

2. Crushing. The grapes are removed from their stems and clusters and are crushed. Traditionally, wine grapes were crushed by human feet using a process called pigeage. Today, that process is seldom used, and most grapes are crushed mechanically. Sometimes, a winemaker may choose to allow some stems to remain when making a red wine in order to have an impact on the wine's development. This is called whole cluster fermentation and can add complexity to the wine's flavor and increase the tannins in the wine. Other times, the winemaker may choose to remove all stems. It depends on what the winemaker wishes to create. If you see the words "Whole Cluster" on the wine label, you can expect the wine to be complex and tannic. The end result of the crushing step in the winemaking process is unfermented grape juice, which is called "must."
3. Fermentation. During this process, yeast converts the sugar in the must into alcohol. Yeast is naturally present, but sometimes more is added at this time to increase the effect. Fermentation is a simple process that requires sugar and yeast. It must take place in an area

with access to air and in the temperature range of 68°F to 86°F for red wine. Yeast cells are bacteria that eat the sugar found in the must. After the yeast eat the sugar, it turns it into both alcohol and carbon dioxide. That is why a fermenting liquid will bubble as it ferments. The bubbling is the carbon dioxide leaving the liquid. The alcohol remains. Wine that starts with juice containing a high sugar level can make a higher alcohol content wine than wine made with low sugar grapes, as the more sugar the yeast has to eat, the more alcohol the yeast can produce. As the yeast eats the sugar, the wine will become less sweet (more dry).

One way to gauge a wine's sweetness is to look at the alcohol content on the label. The higher the alcohol content, the less sweet it is likely to be, as more of the sugar was eaten by the yeast to make alcohol in the fermentation stage of winemaking. Dry wines are usually in the range of 12.5% to 14% Alcohol by Volume (ABV). Off-dry wines are in the range of 11% to 12.5% ABV, and sweet wines are in the range of less than 11% ABV.

Sometimes there is not enough sugar in the grapes for the winemaker to reach the desired level of alcohol. In those cases, sugar can be added to the must. This is called chaptalization. Also, grapes grown in warmer climates can sometimes lack enough acid to make the wine the way that the winemaker wants it to turn out. In that case, the winemaker may add acid to the must at this stage. This is called acidification.

A general rule is that grapes from colder places will be lower in sugar and higher in acid. This is because the cold weather doesn't allow the grapes to ripen as much as warmer climates do. Growers there may need to use chaptalization. German rieslings are famous for needing chaptalization because they are grown in climates so cold that the grapes cannot fully ripen. Whereas grapes grown in warm places will be high in sugar and low in acid. Growers there may need to use acidification.

4. Pressing. In this step, the fermented grape juice is pressed in a wine press so that the liquid is separated from the skins, seeds, and any other solid materials, such as stems. The fact that pressing happens after fermentation will make this wine not white. In the case of rosé wines, also called Blush wines, the wine will be made with dark grapes and have only minimal contact with the skins. Red wines will have significant contact with the skins of dark grapes. Wines made using this method with light grapes are called orange wines. An Orange wine is basically made by using light (white) grapes with a red wine method. Rosé wines are made by using a red wine method with dark grapes but limiting the skin contact in the fermenting stage, and red wines are made by using dark grapes and allowing the skins to remain in contact with the wine until the pressing stage.
5. Aging. This step is also optional. Some wines are ready to be consumed while young, so aging is not required. In fact, aging may hurt some wines. High-quality wines designed to be consumed while young are often less expensive than high-quality wines that are designed to be aged. Therefore, you can often find the best value in a grocery store by purchasing wines that do well when young. However, some wines need to age to improve their drinkability. In this stage, wines may be exposed to oak as a way to soften the tannins and to add structure to the wine. Some wines have to be aged according to the rules that govern their production. For instance, a Chianti Classico wine must be aged at least 12 months before it is bottled. Other wines, such as Beaujolais, are designed to be consumed without any aging at all.

6. Clarification. This stage is optional. There is a current trend toward "natural" or "unfiltered" wines. However, most wines are filtered at this point so that the liquid is clear and free of debris. A cloudy wine may be unfiltered or "natural." Historically, a cloudy appearance in the glass would have been a sign of low quality. However, in recent years, unfiltered wine has become trendy and popular, so some high-quality wines will now be cloudy.
7. Bottling. The final step in the winemaking process is putting the wine into a bottle, closing the bottle with a cork or other covering, such as a screw cap, and labeling the bottle. It used to be the case that only low-quality wines used screw caps. That is not the case today at all. Many very high-quality wines are using screw caps now. In truth, if you set aside tradition and only look at efficiency, screw caps do a better job of sealing a wine bottle than corks do. Corks, being a natural material, can host bacteria that ruin the wine, and they can fail, allowing exposure to air that will ruin the wine. We will talk about "corked wine" later in the book. For now, just know that seeing a screw cap on a bottle of wine these days does not mean the wine is of low quality, like it used to.

To make white wine, the same steps are taken but in a slightly different order. Also, fermentation will take place at a slightly different temperature. White wine ferments at a lower temperature than red wine. White wine ferments between 45°F and 60°F., as opposed to the 68°F to 86°F for red wine. The steps for white wine are as follows:

1. Harvest
2. Crushing (includes destemming)
3. Pressing.
4. Fermenting.
5. Aging
6. Filtering
7. Bottling.

Red vs. White Winemaking Process

RED	WHITE
Harvest	Harvest
Crushing	Crushing
Fermentation	Pressing
Pressing	Fermentation
Aging	Aging
Clarification	Clarification
Bottling	Bottling

Fermentation Temperatures

Red Wine: 68°F to 86°F

White Wine: 45°F to 60°F

As you can see, the difference between the red and white winemaking processes is that white wines are pressed before they are fermented. That means that, unlike red wines, the fermenting must of a white wine will have no contact with grape skins, seeds, or stems. It is this "skin contact" that makes the wine red, so having no skin contact will make the wine white. This means that white wine can be made from dark grapes. For instance, you will find white pinot noirs as well as red pinot noirs. The difference is in the method of winemaking used on the grape, not in the color of the grape itself. Wine that is made with white grapes (also called yellow grapes, or light grapes) that uses the traditional red wine method of skin contact is currently popular and is called "orange wine." Wines made in the red method with dark grapes, but that limit the skin contact, are called rosé or blush wines. Orange wines, as well as Rosé (blush) wines, live in a world between red and white.

Non-Fortified Wine Sweetness Chart by ABV

ABV	Sweetness Level
12.5% or More	Dry
11% to 12.5%	Off Dry
8% to 11%	Semi Sweet
8% or less	Sweet

When shopping for a wine, you will want to know how sweet/dry it is. Most wines do not say "sweet/dry" on the label; instead, the label includes the wine's Alcohol by Volume (ABV). By knowing what ABV level equates to what level of sweetness, one can buy a wine with the desired level of sweetness/dryness.

Some wines are made completely from the same varietal of grape, while other wines are a blend of different grape varietals. A great example of this difference is found when comparing red wines to Burgundy and Bordeaux. Burgundy wines are not mixed; a Red Burgundy is always 100% pinot noir. Bordeaux winemakers are master blenders. A red Bordeaux is a blend of Cabernet Sauvignon, Merlot, and other Red Varietals grown there, such as Malbec. Bordeaux wines that are mostly Merlot come from the Right Bank of the Gironde and Dordogne Rivers, which includes appellations like Pomerol and Saint-Émilion. The Right Bank's clay-rich soils are ideal for merlot, creating wines that are generally richer in plummy fruit flavors and softer in tannins compared to the cabernet sauvignon-dominant wines of the Left Bank.

Different wines are bottled in different types of bottles for a reason. Broadly speaking, wines that have the potential to age well in the bottle are bottled in wine bottles with shoulders; these are often called Bordeaux bottles because wines from Bordeaux are of this sort. This is because when pouring a bottle-aged wine, it is helpful to have shoulders on the bottle to collect sediment when pouring, as sediment forms in wine as it is aging in the bottle. Wines that are intended to be consumed young are commonly bottled in tapered bottles without defined shoulders. These bottles are often called Burgundy bottles for the same reason. These are generalizations, of course, as some young wines are put in bottles with shoulders. It used to be that low-quality wines used twist-top closures, and all high-quality wines used cork. That is no longer the case today. Corks continue to be used because of tradition. Also, due to its porous structure, cork allows tiny amounts of oxygen to enter the wine, which can benefit wines that are particularly tannic and need time in the bottle for those tannins to soften. So, in this case, oxygen – in very small, controlled doses – can be a wine's friend. However, natural cork is also prone to the development of TCA (trichloroanisole). We refer to this as "cork taint" or our wine being "corked," and recognize it by those unpleasant aromas of wet cardboard, musty basement, or mildewy dishcloth. Today, many high-quality winemakers are using twist-off caps on their wine bottles. This is especially true for wines that are not intended to age in the bottle. Wines with cork closures must always be stored on their side so that the cork stays in contact with the wine and does not dry out. Wines with twist-off caps can be stored upright. All wine should be stored out of direct sunlight in a place that is not subject to extreme temperature fluctuations. Ideally, the wine will be kept between 45 and 65 degrees Fahrenheit.

CHAPTER 5

Where Wine is Made

Location. Location. Location. As in real estate dealings, location matters much in winemaking. A wine's location is described in several ways. "Terroir" is a French term referring to the unique set of environmental factors, such as soil, climate, topography, and human tradition, that collectively influence the characteristics of a wine. These factors are interconnected, with elements like soil composition affecting drainage and nutrient availability, while climate and aspect influence sunlight exposure and temperature, all shaping the final taste and quality of the wine.

The climates of wine-growing regions are given on labels:

A "continental climate" is defined by extreme seasonal temperature variations, with hot summers and cold winters. Continental climates are found in large, landlocked regions, primarily in the Northern Hemisphere's interiors of North America, Europe, and Asia. The lack of moderating ocean influence causes temperatures to swing wildly throughout the year, creating a distinct four-season cycle. Additionally, there is great diurnal shift, meaning that the daytime temperature is much hotter than the nighttime temperature.

A "maritime climate," also called an oceanic climate, is characterized by mild, cool summers and winters, a relatively narrow annual temperature range, and consistent, evenly dispersed precipitation. This climate is influenced by the stable temperatures of nearby oceans, resulting in less extreme weather compared to inland continental climates, and is generally found on the western sides of continents in higher middle latitudes, such as Western Europe, the Pacific Northwest of North America, and New Zealand.

A Mediterranean climate features mild, wet winters and hot, dry summers, resulting from stable high-pressure systems in summer. This climate is found in regions like the Mediterranean Basin, coastal California, central Chile, and southwest South Africa.

The term "macroclimate" refers to the overall climate of a region. The term "mesoclimate" refers to the climate of a particular individual vineyard. The term "microclimate" refers to the specific environment in small, restricted spaces such as a single row of vines.

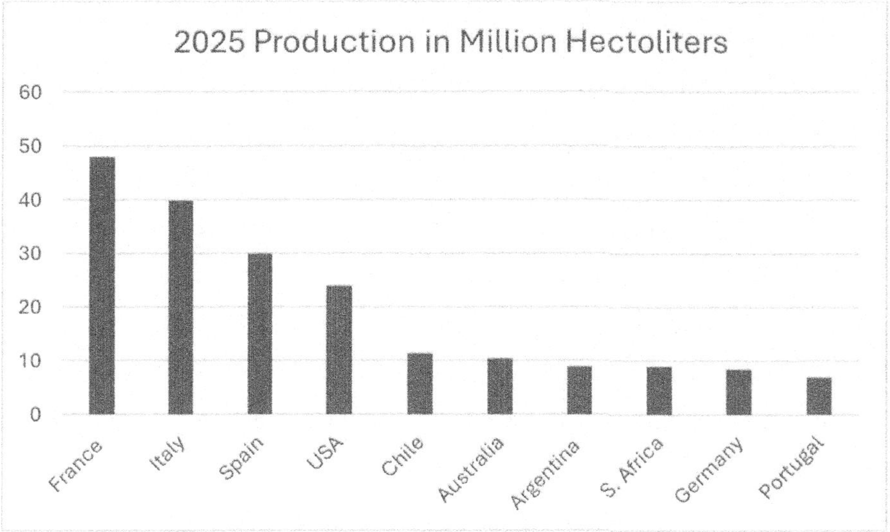

Wine is produced between the 30th and 50th parallels of Latitude, both North and South. Basically, there are two bands of territory around the world where conditions are right for wine production: 30 degrees to 50 degrees north of the Equator and 30 to 50 degrees south of the Equator. Almost all of the world's wine production takes place within these two rings.

Wine-producing areas fall into one of two categories: "Old World" or "New World." A good way to think of this is that if the location was producing wine before Columbus sailed the ocean blue in 1492, the location is "Old World," and if wine production started in the location after that date, the location is "New World."

To confuse things a little bit, Old World wines are often named based on the location where they are made, but New World wines are often named based on the type of grape varietal used to make the wine. In the Old World, each geographic place uses only one (or sometimes a small number) of grape varietals, and a specific geographic place makes only a certain type of wine; that wine is made nowhere else. So, the wine and the place name become synonymous. However, in the New World, any grape variety may be grown in any location, and the same location may produce many different types of wine. This lack of uniformity is often very confusing to wine drinkers. For instance, we call the French wine simply "Red Burgundy," and we then must know that it is made with pinot noir grapes from our own independent study. The varietal will rarely appear on a label of Old-World wines and is rarely mentioned when talking about the wine. We don't say "I had a great pinot noir from Burgundy" because all of the red wine coming out of Burgundy is made from pinot noir grapes. We just say, "I had a great Burgundy." Conversely, a wine made with the same grapes in the United States will not be named after its location. Instead, it will be labeled by its grape varietal. For instance, a wine from the United States would be called a "Pinot Noir" and not an "Oregon." In the case of wines from the United States, we will have to read the label to see where it comes from, and sometimes the label doesn't get very specific. We wouldn't say of an American wine, "This is an Oregon" because there are many types of wine made in Oregon. Instead, we would say "this is a pinot noir from Oregon." This problem was made even more confusing in the early days of American winemaking, when American winemakers often labeled their wines with French location names because they were using the same grape varietal that was grown in those French locations. For instance, in looking at wine labels from the 1940s, one may see wines labeled "California Burgundy." Today, most California winemakers would call that same wine a "California Pinot Noir" or just call it a "Pinot Noir" and write California on the label somewhere. Unfortunately, some American winemakers persist in this bad and confusing naming convention, but not that many any longer. To navigate this complexity, it is important to know which grape varietals are grown in which location in the Old World.

The chart below can help when working with French wines.

Location/Name of Old-World Wine	Grape Varietal	Where the Same Grapes are Used in the Rest of the World
Bordeaux	Cabernet Sauvignon, Merlot, Cabernet Franc, Petit Verdot	USA, Australia, South Africa, Chile, Bulgaria, Romania, Spain, Italy, Lebanon
Burgundy (red)	Pinot Noir	USA, New Zealand, Australia, South Africa
Burgundy (white)	Chardonnay	Australia, New Zealand, USA, South Africa, Chile, Argentina, Spain, Italy, Bulgaria, Hungary
Northern Rhône	Syrah (shiraz)	Australia, New Zealand, USA, South Africa
Alsace	Gewurztraminer, Riesling	New Zealand, Australia, USA
Sancerre	Sauvignon Blanc	New Zealand, Chile, USA, South Africa
Champagne	Chardonnay, Pinot Noir, Pinot Meunier	USA, Australia, New Zealand, South Africa

Here is a similar table for Italian wines that are called by the locations they are made, rather than their grape varietal:

Location/ Old World Wine Name	Grape Varietal	New World Location Grapes Grown
Barolo	Nebbiolo	California, Washington, Oregon, South Africa
Barbaresco	Nebbiolo	California, Washington, Oregon, South Africa
Chianti	Sangiovese	California, Argentina, Australia, Chile
Amarone	Corvina	Limited outside of Italy, Australia, Argentina
Valpolicella	Corvina	Limited outside of Italy: Australia, Argentina
Barbera d'Asti	Barbera	Limited outside of Italy: California
Primitivo	Zinfandel	California

Additionally, the Spanish wine known as Rioja is made of the tempranillo grape.

Generally speaking, wines from warmer climates will have less acid and more sugar, and wines made in cooler climates will have more acid and less sugar. Cooler climate wines with lower natural sugar levels in the grapes are typically lighter-bodied, crisp, with high acidity and lower alcohol content. Whereas grapes grown in warmer climates typically develop more sugar, leading to wines with higher alcohol content, fuller bodies, and riper, fruit-forward flavors. The extended time for grapes to ripen in warm, sunny conditions increases their sugar levels, which yeast converts into alcohol during fermentation. This process also results in lower acidity, making the wine softer and sometimes described as "jammy." Wines made in the New World will be more fruit-forward, and wines made in the Old World will be more subtle and have more minerality.

Top 10 Winemaking Countries

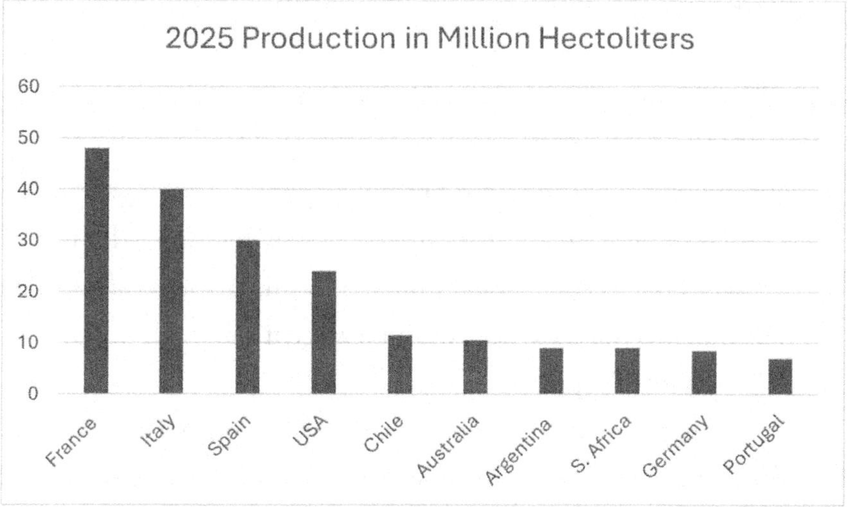

WINES FROM FRANCE

France is the top wine-producing country in the world, producing more than 48 million hectoliters of wine per year. Not only does France lead in quantity, but it also leads in quality. French wine is considered by many to be the best wine in the world, and understandably so. Perhaps no people on earth take their wine more seriously than the French. French wine is heavily regulated and steeped in unbreakable tradition. France has been producing wine continuously since at least Roman times, and today there are 363 uniquely specific wine-growing areas in France. These special areas are called "Appellation d'Origine Contrôlée." Each Appellation d'Origine Contrôlée (AOC) has strict rules governing the types of grapes that can be grown and the winemaking methods that can be used within its carefully defined boundaries. Additionally, within each of the different AOCs, an additional rigid hierarchy of quality designators is often found. This system of organized wine production, which has evolved over the centuries, has been in its current form since 1935. Knowing how French wine is produced and organized can help a person know exactly what to expect from the bottle of wine based on its label. We will now provide a simplified overview of the French system and an overview of key French wine production areas, which will be helpful to the average wine buyer.

General French Wine Quality Levels (Low to High):

1. Vin de France (Wine from France)

   Every wine made in France qualifies for this title, but only 20% of French wine production carries this label, as the remaining 80% qualify for a higher-ranking designation.

2. Wines with Geographic Indication

   This designation means that the wine comes from one of the officially recognized winemaking regions. Thirty percent of all French Wines have this designation.

3. Wines from an Appellation d'Origine Contrôlée (AOC).

   This means that the wine comes not only from one of the 74 officially recognized winemaking regions, but it also comes from a place in that area with specific rules, guidelines, and traditions. Fifty percent of all French wines have this designation.

Within some Appellation d'Origine Contrôlée areas, there are additional levels of quality that wines will be identified with.

BURGUNDY

Wines in the Burgundy Appellation d'Origine Contrôlée can be ordered into one of four levels. The lowest is simply Appellation d'Origine Contrôlée Burgundy, meaning the wine is from Burgundy. Fifty-six percent of wines from Burgundy have this designation. The next step up is the Village designation. Thirty percent of Burgundy wines hold this distinction. That means that the wine comes from a village (area) in Burgundy that is known for making high-quality wine. The next step up is Premier Cru. There are about 600 different Premier Crus in Burgundy, and 12% of

Burgundy wine holds this designation. This means that the wine is from a specific vineyard that is known to be very good. The best Burgundy wines are from one of the 33 Grand Crus. This wine is from the absolute best vineyards in Burgundy, and only 2% of Burgundy wines hold the Grand Cru designation.

Furthermore, there are sub-regions within Burgundy. Those include Chablis, famous for its crisp wine made with chardonnay grapes. Wine from Chablis can be further classified as a Petit Chablis, or one of 40 of Chablis Premier Cru wines, or the best, a Chablis Grand Cru.

Another subregion of Burgundy is Pouilly-Fuissé, famous, like Chablis, for its white wines made from chardonnay grapes. Even though both Chablis and Pouilly-Fuisse are in Burgundy and produce white wine from chardonnay grapes, the wine they produce is significantly different. Pouilly-Fuissé is a rich and complex wine that is often barrel-aged to develop tropical fruit, stone fruit, and toasty notes with a full body. In contrast, Chablis is a mineral-driven, high-acid, unoaked wine known for its lean, crisp, citrusy, and flinty, clean character.

Another subregion of Burgundy is the Côte d'Or. Translated into English, this name means "hillside of gold" because it is so good for making wine. The Cote D'or gets further divided into two main areas. The northern part, called the Côte de Nuits, and the southern part, called the Côte de Beaune. As you can see from the list of Burgundy Grand Crus below, this area is great for wine production.

Grand Cru	Region	Wine style
Chablis Grand Cru	Chablis	White wine
Chambertin	Côte de Nuits	Red wine
Chambertin-Clos de Bèze	Côte de Nuits	Red wine
Chapelle-Chambertin	Côte de Nuits	Red wine
Charmes-Chambertin	Côte de Nuits	Red wine
Griotte-Chambertin	Côte de Nuits	Red wine

Grand Cru	Region	Wine style
Latricières-Chambertin	Côte de Nuits	Red wine
Mazis-Chambertin	Côte de Nuits	Red wine
Mazoyères-Chambertin	Côte de Nuits	Red wine
Ruchottes-Chambertin	Côte de Nuits	Red wine
Bonnes-Mares	Côte de Nuits	Red wine
Clos de la Roche	Côte de Nuits	Red wine
Clos des Lambrays	Côte de Nuits	Red wine
Clos de Tart	Côte de Nuits	Red wine
Clos Saint-Denis	Côte de Nuits	Red wine
Bonnes-Mares	Côte de Nuits	Red wine
Musigny	Côte de Nuits	Red and some white wine
Clos de Vougeot	Côte de Nuits	Red wine
Échezeaux	Côte de Nuits	Red wine
Grands Échezeaux	Côte de Nuits	Red wine
La Grande Rue	Côte de Nuits	Red wine
La Romanée	Côte de Nuits	Red wine
La Tâche	Côte de Nuits	Red wine
Richebourg	Côte de Nuits	Red wine
Romanée-Conti	Côte de Nuits	Red wine
Romanée-Saint-Vivant	Côte de Nuits	Red wine
Corton	Côte de Beaune	Red and some white wine
Charlemagne	Côte de Beaune	White wine
Corton	Côte de Beaune	Red and some white wine
Corton-Charlemagne	Côte de Beaune	White wine
Corton	Côte de Beaune	Red and some white wine
Charlemagne	Côte de Beaune	White wine
Bâtard-Montrachet	Côte de Beaune	White wine
Bienvenues-Bâtard-Montrachet	Côte de Beaune	White wine
Chevalier-Montrachet	Côte de Beaune	White wine
Montrachet	Côte de Beaune	White wine
Criots-Bâtard-Montrachet	Côte de Beaune	White wine

Red wine in Burgundy is made from the pinot noir grape. White wine is made from the chardonnay grape. Burgundy has a higher number of

Appellations d'Origine Contrôlée (AOCs) than any other French region, and is often seen as the most terroir-conscious of the French wine regions. This is in part because pinot noir is a grape varietal that is extremely sensitive to the impacts of terroir. There can be a noticeable difference in wine made with pinot noir grapes that were grown only feet apart. Because pinot noir is a difficult grape to grow and there is strong global demand for the high-quality wine it can produce when the circumstances are ideal, red wine from Burgundy is among the most expensive wines in the world.

BEAUJOLAIS

The Beaujolais Appellation d'Origine Contrôlée is South of Burgundy, and the grape varietal used here is gamay. Wines from Beaujolais often undergo a process called carbonic maceration, where whole uncrushed grapes are fermented in a sealed vat containing a layer of carbon dioxide. This results in fruity, soft, and distinct red wines. These wines have little tannin and are immediately drinkable. Gamay grapes used to be grown in Burgundy alongside pinot noir, but in 1395, Duke Philippe the Bold, to protect the reputation of the region's finer Pinot Noir wines, called gamay a "bad and disloyal" grape. Fearing its high yield and coarse flavors would tarnish Burgundy's image, he ordered all gamay grapes uprooted from Burgundy, never to be grown there again. Gamay found a new home in the Beaujolais region, where it is grown today. Beaujolais wine is organized into three different categories. The lowest being simply Beaujolais, meaning the wine is from the region. The next step up is Beaujolais-Village, meaning the wine is from one of the 38 areas known for making good wine in the area, and the top level is Beaujolais Cru, meaning the wine is from a well-known vineyard. There are 10 Beaujolais Crus, namely: Saint-Amour, Juliénas, Chénas, Moulin-à-Vent, Fleurie, Chiroubles, Morgon, Régnié, Brouilly, and Côte de Brouilly. To confuse matters here, we also have a wine called Beaujolais Nouveau that is different altogether. This is an easy-drinking, simple, young red wine that is released every year on the third Thursday of November, which is right after harvest. It is designed to be consumed right away as a way to celebrate the harvest. It is of much lower quality than the other wines coming from Beaujolais. Sadly, many people have had a glass of Beaujolais Nouveau and been so disappointed in their lackluster experience that they have written off all wines from Beaujolais. Their loss!

BORDEAUX

Bordeaux wines, also referred to as Claret, are organized differently still. There are rules governing the labeling of Bordeaux wines, but unlike in Burgundy, the wines are not organized based on the wine's quality. Instead, the main purpose of Bordeaux's organization system is to differentiate where the wine is from within Bordeaux. All wines from the region will be of the Bordeaux Appellation d'Origine Contrôlée. After that, the distinctions listed on the label tell us more about who made the wine and where the wine is from within Bordeaux, specifically which chateaux or vineyard has produced the wine, than about the wine's desirability. In Burgundy, the wine label is tied to the ground in which the grapes are grown. In Bordeaux, it is tied to the name of the château (winemaker) who made it. We have to know what types of wine are produced in those different areas and what each château is known for to know what to expect from the bottle. Unlike Burgundy wine, Bordeaux wine is mostly blended, and the nature of the blend will change from year to year and from producer to producer. That is one reason there is great fluctuation in wine from year to year, from Bordeaux. Wines from the Right Bank of the Dordogne and Garonne Rivers are blends where the majority of wine in the blend is Merlot. The soil on the Right Bank is mostly clay and limestone. Wines from the Left Bank are blends where the majority of wine in the blend is Cabernet Sauvignon, and the soil has more gravel. The Left Bank's gravelly soil offers excellent drainage and allows the vines' roots to grow deep, forcing them to struggle for nutrients and water. This struggle, combined with the heat-retaining quality of the gravel and how the gravel will reflect the sun to the underside of the growing grapes, helps produce intensely flavored, age-worthy Cabernet Sauvignon-dominant red wines. But in any one year, the percentage of the wine that is Merlot or Cabernet Sauvignon in a Bordeaux blend will change based on things such as crop production. Was it a bad year for Merlot but a good year for Cabernet Franc? If so, expect less Merlot and more Cabernet Franc in that year's blend. A major reason winemakers in Bordeaux take this approach is that it gives them versatility in years of bad harvests. If one grape variety does poorly, the others can just make up a higher percentage of the blend that year, and they can still sell wine. Of course, the goal is always to make the most interesting wine possible by finding "the perfect blend" to bring to market.

On the Left Bank, we find the winemaking areas of Médoc (including Saint-Estèphe, Pauillac, Saint-Julien, and Margaux), Graves (including Pessac-Léognan), and Sauternes. In these areas, many Cabernet Sauvignon and other red grapes are grown to use in blending. The grapes grown for blending include some merlot, malbec, and mostly cabernet franc. A white wine famous from the Left Bank is the dessert wine made in Sauternes. Sauternes wine is made from the semillon grape and is famously very sweet because the winemakers intentionally allow the grapes to experience noble rot (botrytis), which has the effect of making the wine extremely sweet. The Left Bank also makes some dry white wines from the Sauvignon Blanc grape. But by far, they are most famous for their bold red wines.

On the Right Bank are the winemaking regions of Saint Emilion and Pomerol, which make blends that are primarily Merlot-based, with complex character, low tannin levels, and mild acidity. Right Bank wine has intense dark fruit, licorice, chocolate, and spicy flavors. Saint Emilion is home to 800 different wine producers, and Pomerol is home to 900. There is no shortage of good wine in Bordeaux.

LOIR VALLEY

The Loir River is the longest in France. It starts in the center of the country and meanders more than 600 miles to the Atlantic Ocean. The wine regions along its banks have many different microclimates that allow many different types of wines to be produced here. As Bordeaux is most famous for producing red wines, the Loir Valley is most famous for its white wines. Primary grape varietals grown in the Loir Valley are: chenin blanc, cabernet franc, sauvignon blanc, and melon de Bourgogne.

In the Loir Valley is found the Appellation d'Origine Contrôlée of Vouvray, famous for its white wines made in its mineral-rich soil with chenin blanc grapes. Also in the Loir Valley, Savennières and Anjou produce wonderful wines from chenin blanc grapes, but are not as famous for doing so as Vouvray.

But perhaps the most famous Appellation d'Origine in the Loir Valley is Sancerre, which is known for its exquisite Sauvignon Blanc wine. In recent years, demand for this wine has grown so much that prices have increased significantly. This rise in price of Sancerre wine has motivated many lovers of Old-World Sauvignon Blanc to buy wines from the neighboring Appellation d'Origine of Pouilly Fumé, where excellent wines made from sauvignon blanc grapes are also to be found, but at lower prices.

RHONE VALLEY

Located in the Southeast of France, near the border with Italy, the Rhone Valley is home to excellent wine production. It is divided into two parts, the Northern Rhone Valley and the Southern Rhone Valley. In the North, wines made from single varietals dominate production, and the area produces white wines made from viognier, marsanne, and roussanne, as well as red wines made mostly from Syrah. Most wines from this area are oaked. There are 5 distinct growing areas in the Northern Rhone: Côte-Rotie (Syrah/Viognier red blend), Cornas (Syrah red wine only), Condrieu (Viognier white wine only), and Saint Joseph, Crozes-Hermitage, and Hermitage, which all make red wines from syrah with limited amounts of roussanne and marsanne, and also white wines from roussanne and marsanne grapes.

Wines from the Southern Rhone Valley are organized as follows: All wines from the area can be called Côtes du Rhône wines. Wines that are a step up in quality get the label "villages," and the highest rank of wines from the Southern Rhone Valley are called "Single Village Wines." Single Village producers are: Châteauneuf-du-Pape, Gigondas, Vacqueyras, and Tavel.

By far the most famous wine from the Rhone Valley is Châteauneuf-du-Pape. Translated literally as "The Pope's New Castle," it reminds us that from 1309 to 1377, a time known as the Avignon Papacy, the pope lived in France instead of Rome. During this time, he had this area cultivated for wine for his private use. Over time, the pope left, but the wine stayed. The strong red wine is a grenache-based red blend with rich flavors of dark fruit, spices, and earthy notes, often featuring a GSM (grenache, syrah, mourvèdre) combination. The bottles are of thick dark glass and still have the papal seal molded into the glass bottle today. Because of this, a Châteauneuf-du-Pape can be recognized even without the paper label on the bottle.

ALSACE

Alsace is on the border of France and Germany. At different times in history, it has been controlled by either country. Today it is part of France. The wines here show both French and German roots, as is to be expected of this borderland. The region is most famous for its white wines. More than 90% of wine from Alsace is white. But it does produce some Pinot Noir as well. The white wines produced here are riesling, gewurztraminer, muscat, pinot gris, pinot blanc, and sylvaner. Of these, riesling dominates.

CHAMPAGNE

The Champagne region is located in Northern France, about 90 miles North-East of Paris. It is one of the coolest wine-growing regions in the world. The soil is limestone and chalk. This allows roots to dig deep and provides good moisture while also providing good drainage. Three grape varietals are grown here. The only white variety is chardonnay, and the two red varietals are pinot noir and meunier. Most wines from Champagne are a blend of these grapes. What makes wine from Champagne so special is not the variety of grapes grown, but how the wine is made to create a sparkling, rather than still, wine. Multiple processes can be used to make sparkling wine, but only one method is used in Champagne. It is called the Champagne Method, or Traditional Method. (See information in the "Sparkling Wine" section of this book about how Champagne is made.)

WINES FROM ITALY

Italy is the world's second-largest wine producer and the home of some of the world's best wines. There are more than 500 different grape varietals grown in Italy in more than 500 different areas. Winemaking in Italy is uniquely influenced by the region's geographic and political history. Even though Italy is the geographic home of the ancient Roman civilization, Italy as a unified country did not officially exist until 1861. Before that, what we today call Italy was a series of independent regions. Today, the wine of Italy reflects this historic tradition of winemaking as well as this historic geographic and political diversity. Further impacting Italian wine culture is the fact that before modern transportation methods became available, many villages and towns were extremely isolated due to the rough geography of the area. This meant that many small regions, cut off from easy contact with their neighbors due to difficult terrain, developed their own unique winemaking methods and traditions that were very different from the methods and techniques that were developed by other, equally isolated, villages and towns. Additionally, the geography and climate of Italy are not uniform across the country. Temperatures range from cold to hot and from wet to dry. The resulting impact of these factors is a seemingly endless number of different Italian wines.

Today, many different officially recognized regions produce wine, each with distinct characteristics and main grape varietals. Of those, three main regions dominate, namely: 1. Tuscany 2. The Piedmont 3. Veneto. Tuscany is famously home to Chianti, where wine is made mostly from sangiovese grapes. The Piedmont is home to Barolo & Barbaresco, where wine is made from the nebbiolo grape. Veneto is the home of Prosecco, a sparkling wine made from the amarone grape.

Wine quality designators from Italy are different from those in other countries. All Italian wine falls into one of four categories. This category will appear on the wine's label, allowing you to quickly tell into which category of quality the wine falls.

From lowest to highest, the categories are:

1. Vino da Tavola/Table Wine (VdT)

   This is the most basic level of Italian wine. It has no specific regional origin and might be a blend of grapes from various areas.

2. Indicazione Geografica Tipica (IGT)

   This wine is from one specific area. It indicates a higher quality than basic table wine. It must be made from at least 85% grapes from a specified region.

3. Denominazione di Origine Controllata (DOC)

   This wine is from one of Italy's 20 officially recognized regions known to make good wine. Wine in this category is governed by stricter rules than IGT wines, which include specific regulations on grape varieties, aging, production methods, and geographic origin for a particular region.

4. Denominazione di Origine Controllata e Garantita (DOCG)

   The pinnacle of Italian wine classification. The DOCG label is reserved for high-value, high-quality wines that have proven consistent excellence. These wines undergo a government-guaranteed testing process to ensure strict criteria are met, including chemical and sensory evaluation. Fewer than 80 wine areas carry the DOCG label.

About one third of Italian wine carries either the DOC or DOCG label, with another third being called IGT, and the remaining third being VdT.

There are notable exceptions to this system being used as a quality hierarchy. In recent years, several younger winemakers have wanted to do non-traditional winemaking. They may use grape varietals that are not historic to their geographic region, or they may use a new winemaking technique. The wines they make may be of high quality, but are ineligible for their region's higher designation because they do not conform to the traditional rules. Therefore, there are some interesting wines to be found in the Vino da Tavola or Indicazione Geografica Tipica (IGT) categories, but these wines are the exception to the rule. Famously, the currently popular (and very expensive) "Super Tuscan" wines fall into the IGT category for these reasons.

While Italy's official system centers on VdT, IGT, DOC, and DOCG, there are other labels given to wine that are helpful to the consumer. These aren't separate quality levels, but they do give you helpful information about how the wine was made.

They are:

1. Classico: This means the grapes came from the original, historic heart of the wine region. Usually, this means the wine comes from

the highest quality location. Fun note: bottles of Chianti Classico are easy to identify on the store shelf because every one of them has a black rooster on the label!

2. Superiore: Wines with this label may have a fuller body that comes from having a higher alcohol level and have undergone little more aging than wines without this label. They will have good structure.
3. Riserva: As the name would imply, these wines are aged long and are often very smooth and rich. They are made to be savored slowly.
4. Passito: Wines with this label are made from dried grapes, where sugar is highly concentrated, which means they will be sweet.
5. Spumante/Frizzante: If you see these names on a bottle, it means the wine is a sparkling wine. Spumante is fully bubbly, and Frizzante is gently fizzy.

None of these labels impacts the wine's DOC or IGT status; they just give you a few more clues about what to expect in your glass.

Many Italian wines are named and labeled after the geographic region where they are made. For instance, Barolo is a wine from Barolo. It is made with nebbiolo grapes, but nebbiolo won't appear on the label. That is not true of all Italian wines, however. Some Italian wines are labeled to indicate both the grape variety and the location of the wine's origin. For instance, "Barbera d'Alba" is a wine from Alba made from the barbera grape. Here is a chart that will help figure out Italian wines:

Wine Type	Color	Principal Grape(s)			
Amarone	Red	Corvina, others			
Barbaresco	Red	Nebbiolo			
Barbera d'Alba	Red	Barbera			
Bardolino	Red	Corvina, Rondinella, others			
Barolo	Red	Nebbiolo			
Brunello	Red	Sangiovese			
Chianti	Red	Sangiovese, others may be blended into wine in small amounts.			

Wine Type	Color	Principal Grape(s)			
Dolcetto d'Alba	Red	Dolcetto			
Gavi	White	Cortese			
Lambrusco	Red	Lambrusco			
Montepulciano	Red	Montepulciano			
Orvieto	White	Grechetto, others			
Soave	White	Garganega, others			
Taurasi	Red	Aglianico			
Valpolicella	Red	Corvina, Rondinella, others			
Verdicchio	White	Verdicchio			
Vernaccia	White	Vernaccia			
Vino Nobile	Red	Prugnolo (Sangiovese)			

WINES OF SPAIN

With more than 400 native grape varietals, Spain is the world's third-largest producer of wine, from world-renowned reds like Rioja to crisp whites, such as Albariño, and vibrant sparkling Cava. Spain also makes distinct fortified wines, called Sherry.

Like other Old-World countries, Spain has a hierarchical system for grading wine quality. From lowest to highest, those labels are:

1. Vino de la Tierra (VT) ("Wine of the Land"): A step up, this designation is for wines from a specific, demarcated region with distinct local characteristics. The rules are more flexible than for a DO.
2. Vino de Calidad (VC) ("Quality Wine"): A transitional category for regions that are on their way to achieving DO status. A region must be a VC for at least five years before it can apply for DO status.
3. Denominación de Origen (DO) ("Denomination of Origin"): The most common category for Spanish quality wines, encompassing the majority of the country's winemaking regions. DO wines must adhere to specific rules regarding grape varieties, production methods, and yield limits.

4. Denominación de Origen Calificada (DOCa/DOQ) ("Qualified Denomination of Origin"): The highest tier of Spanish wine regulation, reserved for regions with a long history of quality. This designation has the most stringent rules. As of 2024, only Rioja and Priorat (using the Catalan-language DOQ) hold this status.
5. Vino de Pago (VP) ("Estate Wine"): The highest possible classification, awarded to specific, single estates that have unique soil and climate conditions. This is an exclusive classification for exceptional vineyards that produce wines of distinct character and quality.

The major winemaking regions are Rioja, Catalonia, Galicia, and Castilla y León. Rioja is Spain's most famous region, producing elegant, age-worthy red wines primarily from tempranillo grapes. Catalonia is home to Cava sparkling wine and Priorat's bold, concentrated reds. Galicia is known for crisp, aromatic white wines, particularly Albariño from Rías Baixas. Castilla y León includes regions like Ribera del Duero, which are known for dark, rich red wines, and Rueda, known more for white wines. Finally, Andalucía produces the famous fortified wines of the Sherry region.

Key Spanish grape varieties are: 1. Tempranillo, which is a dominant red grape, particularly in Rioja and Ribera del Duero. 2. Garnacha, which is often blended with Tempranillo in reds or used in Priorat wines. 3. Albariño, which is the prominent white grape of the Rías Baixas region in Galicia. 4. Verdejo, which is a white grape from the Rueda region. 5. Macabeo, which is one of the three primary grapes for Cava.

Additionally, the following terms indicating aging periods may be used on wine labels in Spain:

- Crianza: The youngest category, offering fresh and approachable flavors.
- Reserva: A step up in richness and complexity.
- Gran Reserva: The longest-aged category, for a special, slow-savoring experience.

While Spain is famous for producing inexpensive wines, there are also very rare and expensive wines from Spain. Chief among them are wines from Priorat, a mountainous region known for producing some of the world's most powerful and complex red wines with high alcohol and minerality, primarily from garnacha and carinena grapes grown in unique slate soils called "llicorella." Because it is so hard to grow grapes in this terrain, yields are very low, making this wine rare and highly desirable.

WINES FROM THE UNITED STATES

The United States is the world's fourth-largest producer of wine. As might be expected for a country that is young compared to the countries of Europe, the US is a new player in the world of global wine production. Unlike wines from the Old World that are governed by years of tradition and strict laws controlling how wine can be made, there are very few limits as to what a winemaker can do in the United States. Additionally, the United States is a giant country with great geographic variety and many different types of soil and climate. These factors give winemakers great freedom but also make it very hard to know what any particular bottle of American wine will contain. There are no rules or regulations regarding which grape varietals are used or which winemaking methods are allowed. Terms such as "Reserve" or "Select" can be put on any label at the winemaker's discretion, making the words meaningless on labels.

The earliest Europeans to come to America tried to make wine almost as soon as they got here, but they had little success. They could not get European wine grapes to grow here. In the 1500s, French settlers in Florida successfully made wine from the native muscadine grapes. Today, there is at least one winery in every state, and many of them rely on the native muscadine grape, as it is the only grape that will grow in their location. It wasn't until American westward expansion reached California and the Pacific Northwest that large quantities of land, suitable for large-scale, high-quality wine production, were developed in the United States. Most American wine comes from California.

California winemaking regions can be organized as follows: 1. North Coast (Napa Valley, Sonoma County, (including Russian River Valley), Mendocino, Lake County), 2. Central Coast (Santa Barbara County, Paso Robles, Monterey). 3. Central Valley (the state›s primary winegrape-growing area and home to most of the high bulk/low quality wines from the state). In 1976, at the "Judgement of Paris," California's Chateau Montelena's Chardonnay and Stag's Leap Wine Cellars' Cabernet Sauvignon were judged to be the best white and red wines, respectively, in the world, during a blind tasting, establishing California as a world-class source of wine.

Napa Valley and Sonoma are renowned for Cabernet Sauvignon wines. Napa, Sonoma, and Monterey are celebrated for Chardonnay and Pinot Noir. The Russian River Valley area of Sonoma County is home to some of the best Pinot Noir in America. Other notable areas include the Central Coast for Syrah and Merlot, Paso Robles for its variety, including Zinfandel and Syrah, and Santa Barbara for Chardonnay and Pinot Noir wines that are famously fruit-forward.

Washington State is the United States's second-largest wine-producing region, renowned for high-quality Bordeaux-style blends, Riesling, and Merlot wines. Its diverse desert wine country east of the Cascade Mountains offers varied microclimates and soils, fostering growth for many grape varieties. Popular regions include the Columbia Valley, Walla Walla Valley, Red Mountain, and Lake Chelan, with Woodinville serving as a major hub for wineries closer to Seattle.

Many are surprised to learn that New York is the third-largest wine-producing state in the US. Most famous for Riesling from the Finger Lakes region, the state is home to 35,000 acres of vineyards and roughly 450 wineries across six major growing regions. The six major growing areas are: Finger Lakes, Long Island, Hudson Valley, Lake Erie, Niagara Escarpment, and the Champlain Valley.

The state of Oregon ranks fourth in US wine production. Most famous for its Willamette Valley, the state has several different growing regions within the state›s borders that are well-suited to the cultivation of grapes. Commercial wine production began in Oregon in the 1960s. Today, there are more than 1,000 wineries in Oregon, and more than 82 grape varietals are grown in the state.

Ranking 8th in US State wine production, Michigan is an interesting producer of wine. Due to being surrounded by the Great Lakes, it is home to several microclimates. Commercial wine production began in Michigan in 1868 using native varietals, but it did not begin focusing on making dry, quality wine from established winemaking grapes until the 1970s. When Gerald Ford was President of the United States, he served Tabor Hill's 1971 Vidal Blanc at a state dinner in 1974, marking the first time a Midwestern wine was served at a White House state dinner. The wine was a white wine from Tabor Hill Winery in Buchanan, Michigan, and featured subtle, fruity notes with pear and citrus hints.

While every state does now have at least one winery, the largest difficulty found in making wine in the United States outside of the very limited areas where commercial wine production has found to be very good, is that the climate tends to be too warm or too cold for premium grape production, or climates are too extreme, with many days scorching hot and many days freezing cold at the same location throughout the year. Wineries in these areas, forced to use the grapes native to North America, do not produce good wines because of the grapes' relatively high acidity and thick skins. They produce wines that are sour and tart. To overcome this, winemakers often add sugar, making them syrupy and one-dimensional. When looking for wines from the United States, it is best to stick to wines from an area known for good wine production.

From 1920 to 1933, the sale of alcohol was largely prohibited in the United States under the policy known as "prohibition." This caused many US winemakers to pull up their grape vines and grow other things. Prohibition laws allowed individuals to make up to 200 gallons of wine per year for home use. Since most Americans could not grow their own grapes, they would buy grapes from established vineyards via mail order. To accommodate this request, the vineyards had to start growing very thick-skinned grape varietals that could handle being shipped cross-country. This led many of the vineyards that stayed in grape production to shift the varietals they planted to thicker-skinned wines that, while better for shipping, make lower-quality wines than the traditional winemaking varietals that had been planted before. These factors all contributed to the character of the American wine industry today.

No discussion about wines from the United States would be complete without mentioning White Zinfandel. This wine was invented by accident, in California in 1972. Winemaker Bob Trinchero was trying to make a blush wine at the Sutter Home winery, using zinfandel grapes, which traditionally only produce red wines. White wines were gaining in popularity, and Bob thought that if he could make a blush from them, maybe that would be marketable. Something went wrong with the fermentation. Not all of the sugar in the wine was converted into alcohol by the yeast. Usually, when this happens, a winemaker will add more yeast and attempt to restart the process. Bob decided to simply bottle what he had and sell it. It sold like hotcakes. Americans loved the semi-sweet blush wine with very low acidity, low alcohol, and a simple fruity character. It is truly an American wine.

WINES OF CHILE

For being a New World country, Chile has a relatively long history of wine production that began when Spanish invaders planted wine grapes in

Chilean soil in the 1500s. Since that time, Chilean wine production has expanded and matured a great deal. Today, Chile is the world's fifth-largest producer of wine by volume. Chile's wine industry has grown in large part due to the realities of the Chilean economy, where, as a result of low labor and production costs, wines could be produced for a lower cost than in other places. For many years, it was inexpensive to get wine from Chile to the international market, especially the United States, where demand for low-cost wine was high. This cheap Chilean wine continues to fill shelves around the world. Wine that bears no label of geographic origin, other than "Chile" or "Valle Central," is usually of low quality and produced with a focus on cheap quantity.

Since 1994, the following regions of Chile have been recognized as their wine growing areas: 1. Coquimbo Region (Elqui, Limarí, and Choapa Valleys) 2. Aconcagua Region (Aconcagua, Casablanca, and San Antonio Valleys) 3.The large Central Valley Region (Maipo, Rapel, Curicó, and Maule Valleys), and 4. The South Region (Itata, Bío-Bío, and Malleco Valleys).

Generally speaking, wines made in Chile are made to imitate wines found in other places. That said, Chile does produce some very high-quality wines. Finding them can be hit or miss, however.

There is one grape for which Chile is now famous, carménère. Originally from the Bordeaux region of France, Carménère was brought to Chile along with other European grape types. It was found that this grape grows exceptionally well in Chile. Meanwhile, in France, carménère was mostly killed off by the phylloxera epidemic in Europe in the mid-1800s. When France replanted her vineyards after the epidemic, they did so by grafting old varietals onto the rootstock of phylloxera-resistant grape stock imported from the New World. Carménère would not graft, and so it was not replanted. This left Chile as the place for this grape to grow. Carménère is a dry, medium to full-bodied red wine that you cannot mistake. On the nose, you will notice strong aromas of eucalyptus and basil. On the pallet, you find those same flavors, in addition to those of red and black fruits like cherry, plum, and blackberry. Depending on ripeness and winemaking techniques, it can also have smoky, earthy, or tobacco flavors, especially when aged in oak.

WINES OF AUSTRALIA

Australia is huge! It is therefore not surprising that within its borders are many different types of climates and geographic formations. The best place in Australia for wine production is on the southern side of the country.

Australia's officially recognized wine regions, called Geographic Indications (GIs), are structured into zones and sub-regions, with the four major overarching regions being South Australia, New South Wales, Victoria, and Western Australia. Well-known GIs within these states include Barossa Valley and Adelaide Hills (South Australia), Hunter Valley (New South Wales), Yarra Valley (Victoria), and Margaret River (Western Australia).

Australia is famous for its Shiraz (Syrah), which is by far the country's most popular wine and is produced in the Barossa Valley. Australia also produces much Cabernet Sauvignon in the Margaret River region. Tasmania is known for its cool climate and wines made from pinot noir grapes.

Like the United States, Australia lacks strict rules around varietal usage, winemaking technique, and word usage on labels. This makes it very hard to judge the quality of an Australian wine from the bottle. You may just have to drink them to find out!

WINES OF ARGENTINA

Winemaking began in Argentina in the 1500s when the Spanish planted grapes there. Today, Argentina is known for making some of the world's best Malbec wines. Malbec is a French grape from the Bordeaux region that was originally named Cot. It is an ancient varietal and has produced wine for more than 2,000 years. It was brought to Argentina in the 1800s by immigrants from Europe and has thrived there ever since. Most agree that even though the grape is originally from France, it grows better and produces better wine in Argentina than anywhere else in the world, especially in Argentina's Mendoza area. This is because malbec does well in high-altitude areas with a wide diurnal temperature (i.e., hot day, cold night). Here, the grapes produce more acidity than when grown in France. High altitudes also pose a lower risk of diseases and pests, such as phylloxera, which have plagued French Malbec production. Additionally, the devaluation of Argentina's currency in the early 2000s meant that high-quality Argentine wine could be had on the global market at low prices. For many wine drinkers, their first experience with a high-quality wine was when they drank a Malbec from Argentina. This is because, due to the economic realities of Argentina, this high-quality wine was available at a low price point and therefore in grocery store aisles and on wine lists at inexpensive restaurants, where all the other wine offerings at that price point were of lower quality. This is one reason many people today, when asked about their favorite wine varietal, will say "Malbec," as it is one of the highest quality wines available at lower costs. HINT: If you are in a place that only serves lower-cost wines, order the Argentine Malbec from their list; it is likely the highest quality wine they have. When we think of wine from Argentina, we naturally think of Malbec.

But Argentina produces other wines as well, due to its cooler Patagonia wine region, known for producing elegant Pinot Noir and balanced Chardonnay. Notably, these are the same two varietals grown in the Burgundy region of France.

Under Argentine wine laws, if a grape name appears on the wine label, 100% of the wine must be composed of that grape variety. In addition to Malbec, Pinot Noir, and Chardonay, wines in Argentina are made from torrontés (its signature white grape), bonarda, cabernet sauvignon, and syrah.

WINES OF SOUTH AFRICA

Wine production came to South Africa in the 1600s when the Dutch set up a supply depot there to re-stock their world-traveling trade ships. In order to have wine to stock up their ships when they stopped to resupply, the Dutch planted vineyards in South Africa, and wine has been growing well there ever since. Today, many grapes are grown in South Africa, and chief among them is Pinotage, which is a cross between Pinot Noir and Cinsaut created in South Africa in the 1920s. This dark red wine is South Africa's most famous wine and is similar to a Shiraz. South Africa also produces a sparkling wine, using the traditional Champagne method, which is called Cap Classique. Originally, South Africa's sparkling wines were made from chenin blanc grapes, but now, most Cap Classique wines are produced from the three classic Champagne varieties, chardonnay, pinot noir, and pinot meunier. The country's primary wine-growing areas are centered in three major areas. First, the Western Cape, which includes the coastal region with districts like Stellenbosch, Paarl, Franschhoek, and Constantia. Second, the Breede River Valley, and finally the Cape South Coast (which includes Walker Bay and Elgin. Other, less popular designated wine regions include the Klein Karoo, Olifants River, the Eastern Cape, and the Northern Cape. These regions offer diverse climates and terroir, producing distinct styles of wine, from bold reds and whites in the warmer coastal areas to elegant cool-climate wines in the south.

WINES OF GERMANY

Germany is among the northernmost wine-producing places in the world, and wine production in Germany dates to Roman times. Most of

Germany's wine production takes place in the Western part of Germany along the Rhine River and its tributaries. Germany's most prominent white grape is riesling, and its most prominent red grape is pinot noir, which goes by the name spätburgunder in Germany. Due to the climate, German wines are famous for being highly acidic. Rieslings can range in scope from dry to sweet. German regulations categorize wine by the amount of sugar in the grape juice prior to fermentation. This system does not necessarily determine if a wine is sweet or not because all of the sugar could be consumed during fermentation (making the wine dry and higher in alcohol) or fermentation can stop before all of the sugar is consumed (making the wine sweeter and lower in alcohol). However, it is a helpful guideline. The chart from least to most sugar is below:

Name				Minimum ABV
Kabinett				7%
Spätlese				7%
Auslese				7%
Beerenauslese, Eiswein				5.5%
Trockenbeerenauslese				5.5%

In Germany, dry wines are called "Trocken." Off-dry wines are called "Halbtrocken," semi-sweet wines are called "Lieblich," and sweet wines are called "Sub."

PORTUGAL

Portugal is the world's tenth-largest wine-producing country, largely because of its production of fortified wine called "Port," which is discussed in detail in the fortified wine section of this book. Like many Old-World countries, Portugal has been producing wines since the days of the Roman Empire.

Portuguese wines, similar to Spanish wines, include the white grape variety alvarinho, which is called Albariño in Spain. Portugal's wine, called "Tinta Roriz," goes by the name Tempranillo in Spain. The Portuguese wine, Aragonez, shares similarities with Spanish reds like those from Rioja. Additionally, the Portuguese red grapes, touriga nacional and touriga franca, often found in the Douro region, produce wines with bold, complex profiles similar to Spanish Rioja and Ribera del Duero.

NEW ZEALAND

Wine production in New Zealand began in the 1800s. Today, wine is produced in several distinct winegrowing regions. The country's elongated island shape produces considerable regional variation from north to south. New Zealand wine is usually produced and labelled as single varietal wines, or if blended, winemakers list the varietal components on the label. That said, its most famous wine, Sauvignon Blanc, mostly comes from its Marlborough area. Also from Marlborough comes its dense, concentrated Pinot Noir. Hawke's Bay is the oldest wine-growing region in the country. The area is best known for its red blends and also for its Chardonnay.

CHAPTER 6

Brief Overview of Common Varietals

WHITE GRAPES

Varietal	Grown	Used in Blends?	Acidity	Notes
Alberino	Spain, Portugal	No	High	Floral notes, dry medium-bodied can be oaked or unoaked
Chardonay	France (and almost everywhere else, too)	Yes	Med-High	Very versatile, can range from crisp unoaked from Chablis to buttery and oaked from CA
Chenin Blanc	France, South Africa, New Zealand, the Americas,	Yes	High	Can be oaked or unoaked, dry to sweet
Gerwerstiminer	France, Germany, and some New World			
Muscato	Italy, France, Germany, New World	Yes	Low-Med	
Pinot Grigio/ Gris	Cool climates, Germany, France, USA		High	Can range from sweet to dry, unoaked, light to full body,
Riesling	Cool moderate climate, France, Italy (most places)	Yes	med-high	Young, usually unoaked, light-bodied, simple wine

Varietal	Grown	Used in Blends?	Acidity	Notes
Sauvignon Blanc	France, New Zealand, USA (many places)	Yes - but not often	High	Aromatic, early drinking, great variation between Old/New world examples
Semillon	France (Sauternes)	Yes - but not often	Med – High	Often, a dessert wine when not blended. Famous from Sauternes

Red Grapes

Varietal	Where Grown	Blended?	Acidity	Notes
Gamay	France,	Yes, but rare	Med-High	Famous from Beaujolais
Nebbiolo	Italia	Yes, but not usually	High	Notable wines: Barolo, Barbaresco, Roero Gattinara, Ghemme. Can be oaked or unoaked
Pinot Noir (Germany: Spatburgunder)	France, New World	Very Rarely	Med-High	Famous from Burgundy, very sensitive to terroir and hard to grow
Sangiovese	Italia	Yes	High	Famous from Chianti
Syrah (Shiraz)	France, global	Yes	High	
Barbera	Italia	Yes	High	
Cabernet Sauvignon	France (global)	Yes	High	Famous from Bordeaux Left Bank, now global
Carménère	Chile/France	Yes	high	Originally from France, now Chile's most notable wine
Corvina	Italia	Yes	Med-High	
Grenache	Spain/France (global)	Yes	Low-Med	

Varietal	Where Grown	Blended?	Acidity	Notes
Malbec (Cot)	France, Argentina	Yes	High	Originally from France, now Argentina's most notable wine
Merlot	France (global)	Yes	Med	Wine is famous for having medium traits and plum flavor. From Bordeaux Right Bank
Petite Sirah	France, USA	Yes	Med-High	Big red wine with high tannin
Pinotage	South Africa	Yes	Low	Blend of pinot noir and cinsault grapes invented in South Africa in the 1920s.
Tempranillo	Spain	Yes	Med-High	Spain's most famous wine
Zinfandel (Primitivo)	Italia, USA	Can be, but rare	Med-High	Big red wine. Originally from Italy, now famously a California wine. This grape also makes White Zinfandel, which is a semi-sweet blush wine.

CHAPTER 7

Sparkling Wine

Sparkling wine can be made in different ways. Each way has advantages and disadvantages. Here is a brief overview of those ways and the wines they make.

1. Champagne Method

   This method is also called the Traditional Method or Cap Classique method. As the name implies, it is the method used to make Champagne. This method is also used in Spain to make Cava, in South Africa to make a sparkling wine called Cap Classique, and in Germany to make a sparkling wine called Sekt. The advantage of wine made in this system is that the wine comes out clear and tasting of bread/dough from long exposure to the lees (yeast) during in-bottle secondary fermentation. The disadvantage of this method is that it is time-consuming and expensive. In addition to the distinctive aroma and taste of bread, the bubbles (called beads) in wine made with this method tend to be smaller than those in wines made with other methods. Tiny bubbles also rise more slowly, and so the wine sparkles for longer in the glass. This makes sparkling wines made in the Champagne style the most suited to be served in a traditional wine glass, instead of a flute glass, which concentrates the bubble flow more than an open glass does. It is said by many who enjoy sparkling wine that the smaller the bubble, the better the wine.

Champagne is made with chardonnay, pinot noir, pinot meunier, or a blend thereof. While other grapes are permitted in the Champagne region, such as pinot gris, pinot blanc, arbane, and petit meslier, they are used very rarely and make up a tiny fraction of the total vineyard planting. Champagne must be aged for a minimum of 15 months before release, with non-vintage (NV) Champagne requiring 12 of those 15 months to be on the lees (where the wine is exposed to the yeast in the bottle, taking up bread-like flavor). Vintage Champagne has stricter rules, needing a minimum of three years of aging on the lees before release.

Cava is usually made using macabeo, xarel·lo, and parellada grapes. Other authorized grapes can also be used, including chardonnay and malvasia, as well as the red grapes garnacha, monastrell, pinot noir, and trepat, which are used to create rosé wines. Cava has four aging categories. They are, from shortest to longest aging time: A. Cava de Guarda (at least 9 months aging on the lees), B. Reserva (at least 18 months aging on the lees), C. Gran Reserva (at least 30 months aging on the lees), and the top tier, Cava de Paraje Calificado, which requires at least 36 months of aging on the lees. These aging categories determine a Cava's complexity, with longer aging periods leading to more nuanced flavors like toast, nuts, and brioche.

South Africa's Cap Classique wines are made from chardonnay, pinot noir, pinot meunier, chenin blanc, or a combination thereof. Cap Classique wines must age on their lees for a minimum of 12 months after the secondary fermentation in the bottle before disgorgement. While this 12-month minimum is the regulation set by the Cap Classique Producers' Association (CCPA), many top producers age their wines for longer to achieve more complex flavors.

Sekt is usually made from riesling, pinot blanc, pinot gris, and pinot noir, or a blend thereof. Other grapes, such as chardonnay and silvaner, are also used, particularly for high-quality versions. For Rosé Sekt, pinot noir is the primary grape. Sekt is often made from grapes imported into Germany. There is no aging requirement for this wine. However, if the wine is made from German grapes, it is then labeled as German Sekt and must age a minimum of 9 months on the lees to gain the designation "Winzersekt" wine, called "VDP Sekt," which requires at least 15 months of lees aging, and wine called "VDP Grosse Lage Sekt" requires a minimum of 36 months of lees aging.

Additionally, there are some makers of sparkling wine using the traditional method in the United States and other places, but since no regulations exist in those places to govern the wine's production methods, they cannot be known or spoken of in general.

All wines made using the Traditional Method are made using the following steps:

A. Make the base still wine. Grapes are pressed quickly and gently, and the base wine is very light in color. Fermentation can take place in either oak barrels or in stainless-steel tanks.
B. Blend the wines. This is called creating the Cuvee. The winemaker will blend the base wines to create the desired wine.
C. Secondary fermentation. This creates the bubbles. The base wine is bottled with a mixture of yeast and sugar, which is called the "liqueur du triage." The bottle is sealed with a crown cap. The yeast then eats the sugar and emits carbon dioxide, which is trapped inside the bottle, making the wine bubbly.
D. Autolysis. The wine is rested "on the lees." This means that the wine is stored so that the yeast/sugar combination, called the "lees," has contact with the wine. This exposure to yeast will

give the wine a distinctive bread-like taste and smell. By law, all Champagne must spend at least 12 months on the lees as part of a minimum 15-month total aging process.

E. Remuage. In this stage, the sediment is removed. Each bottle is gradually turned to move the lees into its neck. The wine must sit in this position long enough for all of the yeast to drift down to the bottom of the bottle in the neck and have none left in the rest of the wine. This usually takes a couple of months.

F. Degorgement. In this stage, each bottle's neck is frozen in an ice bath, the cap is removed, and the frozen yeast (lees) is removed.

Dosage. A mixture of wine and sugar is then added to the bottle to determine the wine's final level of sweetness, and therefore, style of champagne.

The Dryness of Champagne is labeled using the following system

Bone Dry	Brut Nature
Very Dry	Extra Brut
Dry	Brute
Off Dry	Extra Dry
Semi Sweet	Sec
Sweet	Demi Sec
Very Sweet	Doux

2. The Tank Method

The Tank Method is also called the Charmat Method or the Martinotti Method. It was invented by the Italian, Federico Martinotti, and further developed by the Frenchman, Eugène Charmat.

For Prosecco, the sparkling wine from Italy, the Tank Method is famously used. Prosecco is made using glera grapes and has no aging requirement. Generally, Prosecco is made to be consumed while young and fresh, with an ideal window of consumption generally being within 1-2 years of bottling. However, some Prosecco Superiore DOCG wines can be aged for longer, with a minimum release after 18 months, and some high-quality or vintage bottlings may be aged for up to seven years or more.

The process for making sparkling wine with the Tank Method is as follows:

A. Make the base still wine. Grapes are pressed quickly and gently, and the base wine is very light in color. Fermentation can take place in either oak barrels or in stainless-steel tanks
B. Add yeast and sugar to the wine while
C. Move the wine into a sealed stainless-steel vat
D. Secondary fermentation will occur in the tank, and since the tank is sealed, the CO2 will stay in the wine since it can't escape into the air
E. Pump the wine through a filter so that the lees are removed from the wine
F. Bottle the wine under pressure so the bubbles don't escape.

The advantage of this method is that it is much easier, faster, and therefore, less expensive than the Champagne Method, since all the work is done in one large tank, instead of in individual bottles. The downside is that the wine has less exposure to the lees and is therefore less flavored by the yeast. The bubbles are also larger and dissipate faster in the glass, making a flute glass a good serving choice for wine made with the tank method.

3. The Asti Method

The Asti Method is a variation of the tank method designed to create sweeter wines. This is used in Northern Italy to create low-alcohol sweet sparkling wines with the Muscato grape. These wines are not aged. Here are the steps for the Asti Method:

A. Start with non-fermented grape juice of the Moscato grape
B. Partially ferment it inside a pressurized tank that is sealed to retain the CO_2.
C. Stop fermentation before all of the yeast is consumed, thus making a sweet wine with low alcohol content.
D. Filter the wine to remove yeast
E. Bottle the filtered wine under pressure

4. The Pétillant Naturel Method

   The oldest method used to make sparkling wine is starting to come back into fashion. The method for making this wine is called the Pétillant naturel method or ancestral method, and wines made with this method are often called "Pét-nats."

   Rather than induce a second fermentation in the bottle to create the bubbles, as the Champagne method does, makers of pét-nat wines simply bottle the wine before the initial fermentation has ended. The result is softly fizzy, sometimes lightly sweet from residual grape sugars, usually hazy with unfiltered yeast particles, and typically sealed with a crown cap instead of a cork. These wines are made of many different grape varietals and are not designed to be aged. If left in the bottle too long, the wine will lose its fizz. The wine will be cloudy when served, as the lees are never removed during the winemaking process. The wine will also have a complex flavor from the exposure to the yeast.

5. Carbonation Injection Method.

   The cheapest way to make a sparkling wine is to inject CO_2 into the wine in the same way that CO_2 is injected into soda pop. This method is called the Injection Method. It is used in places where there are no regulations governing how wine must be made, such as in the United States. It is used because it is the cheapest way to make a sparkling wine. It imparts no flavor or aroma. Low-cost sparkling wines come from the New World, which often uses this method. Wine made with this method is best served with orange juice to make a mimosa, rather than consumed directly.

CHAPTER 8

Fortified Wines

Fortified wines are wines to which a distilled spirit, most often a brandy (which is itself distilled wine), has been added to increase their alcohol content and preserve them. The addition of the spirit, which is done either during or after fermentation, affects the wine's flavor profile and often results in a higher residual sugar content. Examples of fortified wines include Port, from Portugal, Sherry, from Spain, Madeira, from the island of Madeira, and Vermouth. Vermouth was originally made in France and Italy and is now made around the world. Today, it is mostly used as an ingredient in cocktails. We will now look at the fortified wines, Port, Sherry, and Madeira, in greater detail.

PORT

Port is a wine steeped in tradition. One port tradition involves a host placing the decanter to their right and passing it to the left, moving clockwise around the table until it returns to the host. This tradition is called "port-to-port" because the port is moving to the port (nautical term for left) and originated in the British Royal Navy. It ensures continuous circulation and equal opportunity to enjoy the wine. If the decanter stalls with one guest, a polite, indirect reminder is to ask the person where the wine is stalled: "Do you know the Bishop of Norwich?" If that alone is not enough to remind him to circulate the port, then the person says, "He's a wonderful fellow, but he always forgets to pass the port." It is said that this tradition originated with Bishop Henry Bathurst of Norwich (1805-1837), who would often fall asleep after dinner, causing the port to stop moving around the table. Port is produced in the Douro Valley of northern Portugal, where wine has been produced for thousands of years. In the 1700s, the area was officially declared a winemaking region by the English. Why do the English have such a connection to wines from Portugal? In the 1700s, England was frequently at war with France and on bad terms with other European winemaking countries, which limited their supply of wines from those places. The English began to look for other wine trading partners because England is not a great place to grow grapes. They found their partner in the winemakers of Portugal, and the English developed a taste for Port. Additionally, during this time, Britain ruled the waves, and fortified wines did well on ships because a fortified wine would not spoil like a traditional wine. Port, therefore, developed a following among sailors, and England in the 1700s had many sailors. Port is typically a sweet red wine, often served with dessert, although it also comes in dry, semi-dry, and white varieties.

The main grapes used to make red port include touriga franca, tinta roriz, tinta barroca, touriga nacional, tinto cão, and tinta amarela. White Port is made with grapes like malvasia fina, gouveio, rabigato, and viosinho.

White port is much less common than red port and offers a range of flavors, from fresh and young aperitifs to rich and complex wines aged in wood for up to 40 years. An impressive drink on its own, it is often used in cocktails like the porto tónico (white Port and tonic). It is made in small quantities by about 30 producers. It can range from mostly dry to intensely sweet.

Red port falls into two main categories, namely Ruby or Tawny. Ruby ports are organized into additional types, including "ruby," "vintage," and "late bottle vintage (LBV)." Ruby ports are more ruby red in color, and Tawny ports have a tawny brown color. As for flavor, both have a sweet taste. However, Ruby ports have more of a fruity, berry flavor, and Tawny ports tend towards a nutty, caramel flavor.

Ruby and Tawny ports start the same way in the production process. Grapes are harvested and undergo a very short maceration and fermentation process in which producers foot tread the grapes or use special fermentation equipment in order to gently extract as much color and flavor as possible from the grapes before adding a grape spirit to the wine. The high alcohol in the spirit immediately halts the fermentation process, leaving a wine that is high in alcohol, yet still has residual sugar. This is the secret to the unique quality of fortified wines. Because distilled grape spirit is added, it will have a high alcohol level, but because the natural fermentation of the wine itself was halted early, it remains sweet since the yeast did not eat all of the sugar. This gives a sweet wine with an alcohol content so high that the wine will not spoil as fast as normal wines do. From there, the wines are designated into the Ruby or Tawny category.

Ruby ports are aged in large oak casks, which allows the wine to keep the youthful ruby color and all of the fresh fruity flavors, because the wine has very little contact with the oak and oxygen. Tawny ports are aged in small oak barrels, which causes the wine to change color and flavor because of the close contact with the oak and greater surface contact with oxygen.

Typically, Ruby ports match extremely well with chocolate, especially with a raspberry sauce or mixed berries. They also pair well with full-flavored or soft-ripened cheese, such as a Stilton or Gorgonzola. Tawny ports match up well with cheesecake, apple pie, or a simple bowl of fresh walnuts, as well as cheeses that are dry or slightly salty, such as Parmigiano Reggiano or an aged goat cheese.

Basic Ruby Port:

There are six types of Ruby Port, with those labeled as simply Ruby Port being the most basic. These wines, often bulk-produced, are made from a blend of younger wines from many vintages. They are easy-drinking, inexpensive, sweet wines; tasty, but not something to bring to dinner with the in-laws.

The prestigious Vintage Ports are on the opposite end of the Ruby Port spectrum. These are elegant wines. They are dark purplish red in color and have vibrant acidity to balance their sweetness. They are made from top-quality grapes and are only produced in the very best years. A Vintage Port can only be made in years where the grape harvest produces extremely high-quality grapes. These wines spend no more than two years in barrels before being bottled and are intended to be cellared by the buyer. These special wines can be left to sit for decades and will gain complexity. There was a tradition among English aristocrats of buying port when their son was born and drinking it with him when he turned 21 years old. While many people wouldn't dare drink a Vintage Port until it's had at least 15 to 30 years of aging, younger examples (up to 5 years old) can also be wonderfully tasting. They're a different animal than the longer-aged versions, and are dominated by ripe red and black fruit flavors and have strong tannins. Port that is at least 15 years old is full of flavors, such as dried fruit (particularly figs), black cherry, honey, pepper, spice, almonds, and even hints of tea leaves and tobacco.

A classic food pairing with Vintage Port includes Stilton or other richly flavored cheeses accompanied by dark chocolate, figs, and walnuts. For dessert, try Vintage Port with anything chocolate.

Between simple Ruby Port and Vintage Port, there are four other types of Ruby Port. From lowest to highest quality, they are:

A. Reserve Ruby Port is a step up from simple Ruby Port, made from better fruit and with more stringent standards.

B. Crusted Port is bottled unfiltered, leaving a sediment (crust) that forms in the bottle. This full-bodied style is similar to Vintage Port but at a much lower price point.

C. Late Bottled Vintage (LBV) is similar to Vintage Port in that it is from a single year and made of high-quality fruit. Unlike Vintage, it is bottled after a longer time in barrels, for four to six years, and it's produced yearly, not just in the most outstanding years.

D. Vintage Single Quinta is the most similar in style to Vintage Port, except that it originates from a single estate (called a quinta), whereas Vintage Port can be sourced from a variety of quintas.

Like Vintage Port, Tawny Port is a connoisseurs' wine. Tawny Port maintains a moderate to high acidity level with a sugar level that is not too high, creating balance. In contrast to the powerful, fruit-forward Vintage Port, Tawny is aged before you buy it and is not meant to be cellared further. It is released in 10-, 20-, 30-, and 40-year-old versions, with the age referring to time spent in wood. The age on the wine bottle is the average age of the grapes in that bottle. Since it is made from a blend, some of the wine in the bottle will be older and some will be younger than the age on the bottle, it being the average age of the wine. 10-year-olds show youthful fruitiness, whereas 20-year-olds offer more complexity and a lively freshness. 30- and 40-year-olds tend to be richer and sweeter with a more unctuous texture. Tawny Port offers more subtle flavors, such as caramel, peanut brittle, dried fruits (apricots, dates, raisins, prunes), nutmeg, chocolate, and walnuts. With its nutty nuances, Tawny Port pairs naturally with nut-based desserts like pecan pie and almond biscotti. It also partners well with savory items such as a charcuterie board of salamis and thinly sliced hams, Pecorino cheese, olives, dried prunes and apricots, potato chips, and nuts. The alcohol by volume (ABV) of port wine typically ranges from 19% to 22%.

SHERRY

Sherry is a fortified wine made in Spain. It is produced in a variety of styles, from sweet to dry, and is made primarily from the palomino grape, ranging from light versions similar to white table wines, such as Manzanilla and Fino, to darker and heavier versions that have been allowed to oxidize as they age in barrel, such as Amontillado and Oloroso. Sweet dessert wines are also made from pedro ximénez or moscatel grapes, and are sometimes blended with Palomino-based sherries.

Perhaps the most unique thing about sherry is the system by which it is aged. The system is called the Solara System. Solara means ground, and it refers to the fact that the wine is aged in barrels stacked on the ground in a rotational system. The Solera System is a fractional blending and aging process that uses a tiered system of barrels (solera and criaderas) to ensure consistency and complexity in sherry wines across many vintages. Wine is drawn from the oldest barrels (the solera) for bottling, then these are replenished with wine from the next youngest tier (a criadera), and so on, with the youngest tier being topped up with new wine from the current harvest. This continuous cycle allows for the creation of a consistent house style while imparting the rich, complex character of a living, evolving system over time, and is the reason sherry is a non-vintage wine.

Sometimes the barrel in the Solera System is not filled all the way; this allows a layer of yeast to form at the top of the liquid. This layer is called the "Flor." Sherry wine, such as Fino and Manzanilla, is made using this method. This protective yeast layer prevents oxidation, resulting in light, dry, fresh wines with characteristic nutty, almond, or bread-like aromas and flavors. Other sherries are aged without flor, such as Oloroso, which is aged oxidatively, leading to a richer, darker, and more complex wine.

Sweet sherries include pedro ximénez (PX), moscatel, as well as sherries labeled as Cream and Medium sherries, which are made either from late-harvested and dried sweet grapes or by adding sweet grape syrups to a dry base wine to retain or add sweetness. Dry sherries include Fino (has floor, bread flavors, nutty and complex), Manzanilla (has flor, bread flavors, nutty and complex), Amontillado (darker than Fino sherry, but lighter than Oloroso), Oloroso (rich, full body, highest alcohol content), and Palo Cortado (aromatic refinement of Amontillado, with the body and structure of Oloroso, which are typically made from dry palomino grapes.)

The Alcohol by Volume (ABV) of sherry ranges from 15% to 22%, with specific types having minimum requirements, such as Fino and Manzanilla, requiring at least 15% ABV, while Amontillado, Palo Cortado, and Oloroso must be at least 17% ABV.

MADERIA

Wine has been made on the island of Madeira since at least the 1600s. Originally, Madeira wine was fortified to help preserve it for transport. The wine made its way around the world, sloshing around in wooden barrels, in the holds of sailing ships. When faster ships were invented and the Maderia was delivered faster, it was noted that the quality had decreased. It was then realized that the process of transporting the wine in the sloshing ship was adding to the wine's flavor profile. Today, wine is aged in a way to simulate the experience of transit in a sailing vessel before it is bottled. Maderia wine was much enjoyed in colonial North America and was a favorite of American founding fathers, such as Thomas Jefferson, John Adams, and Benjamin Franklin. It was commonplace in 1700s America to serve a glass of Madeira wine with a dish of walnuts at the conclusion of a dinner. Maderia was known as "America's wine," and when Americans would go to Europe and drink good non-fortified wines for the first time, they were often shocked at the difference.

Approximately 85% of Madeira is produced with the red grape, negra mole. The four major white grape varieties used for Madeira production are (from sweetest to driest) malvasia, bual, verdelho, and sercial.

Madeira wine is made using one of two methods: the "Canteiro" Method, a traditional, slow aging process in warm attics for premium wines, and the "Estufagem" Method, a quicker, heated process for younger wines, using stainless steel tanks with hot water jackets. Both processes involve oxidation and heat to create tertiary aromas and flavors of spices, nuts, and dried fruits, contributing to the wine's extraordinary longevity and complex bouquet. These methods replicate how the wine was aged during transit in the days of sail.

All Madeira must be aged at least 3 years before bottling. The sweetness level of a Madeira wine will be labeled as follows

Dry or Extra Dry (Seco)	50-60g/l of sugar; extra dry is less than 20 grams. All wines are made with sercial
Medium Dry (Meio Seco)	60-80g/l. All wines are made with verdelho and some terrantez
Medium Sweet or Medium Rich (Meio Doce)	80-100g/l. All wines are made with boal and some terrantez
Sweet or Rich or Full Rich (Doce)	

Like other fortified wines, Madeira is 15% to 20% ABV.

CHAPTER 9

Wine Faults

"Faults" in wine are undesirable and unpleasant aromas, flavors, or visual characteristics that arise from improper winemaking or storage conditions. Examples include: 1. Cork Taint (it is said that the wine is corked). 2. Oxidation 3. Reduction 4. Volatile acidity (vinegar) 5. Brettanomyces (horse blanket) 6. Heat damage (cooked fruit).

Here are some common wine faults and their characteristics:

- **Cork Taint (TCA)**: Caused by a chemical compound (TCA), it results in a musty or moldy smell, often described as wet cardboard or a damp cellar.
- **Oxidation**: When wine has too much exposure to oxygen, it loses its fresh fruit flavors, develops a dull color (brownish for reds, orangey for whites), and can smell like bruised apples or honey.
- **Reduction**: The opposite of oxidation, reduction occurs when a wine lacks sufficient oxygen. It can produce aromas of rotten eggs, burnt rubber, or garlic. Sometimes decanting can help.
- **Volatile Acidity (VA)**: An excessive amount of acetic acid can give the wine a pungent, vinegar-like smell or a sharp, nail-polish-remover aroma.
- **Brettanomyces ("Brett")**: A type of yeast that can infect wine, producing undesirable aromas, such as band-aids and medicinal notes.
- **Heat Damage**: Storing wine at high temperatures or with excessive fluctuations can lead to a dull, "cooked fruit" or jammy aroma.

- **Lightstrike**: Intense exposure to light can cause delicate white wines to develop a "wet wool" or "wet cardboard" aroma.

How to Identify a Fault:

A. **Look**: Check for changes in color, such as the browning of a red wine or the orangey hue of a white wine.

B. **Smell**: Many faults are detected through smell. Look for aromas that are out of place or unpleasant for the wine's expected style.

C. **Taste**: If the wine tastes off or unbalanced, it may be a sign of a fault.

CHAPTER 10

Fun Wine Tasting Exercises

EXERCISE ONE: SAUVIGNON BLANC

Wines: Sancerre, Pouilly-Fumé, New Zealand Sauvignon Blanc

Price: Expect to pay $35 for the Sancerre, $35 for the Pouilly-Fume, and $15 for the New Zealand Sauvignon Blanc.

Process: Pour each wine into a glass and set them next to each other in the order described above. Compare and contrast the coloration. Next, smell the wines and note the differences. Then, take a drink of each wine in the assigned order. Note how the same grape, sauvignon blanc, creates different wines based on where the wine grapes are grown and where the wine is made. Sancerre is a Loire Valley Sauvignon Blanc characterized by high acidity, citrus, and fresh grass flavors, while Pouilly-Fumé offers a more restrained, mineral-driven profile with subtle smoky, flinty, or stone fruit notes, often on a broader, more rounded texture. The key differences stem from their terroir, with Pouilly-Fumé's soils typically containing more silex (flint), giving it the characteristic "fumé" or smoky aroma. The wine from the New World will be very different. New Zealand Sauvignon Blanc from Marlborough is known for its intense, fruit-forward profile with tropical notes of passion fruit, gooseberry, and zesty grapefruit, complemented by herbaceous characteristics like cut grass and bell pepper. The key difference is Sancerre's refined complexity versus New Zealand's bold, tropical intensity, driven by distinct terroirs and climate.

EXERCISE TWO: PINOT NOIR

Wines: Red Burgundy, Russian River Pinot Noir, inexpensive Pinot Noir

Price: Expect to pay between $30 and $50 for a bottle of red burgundy, $40 for a bottle from the Russian River Valley, and then buy the cheapest pinot noir you can find, $10.00.

Process: Look at, smell, and drink the wines in the order described. Note how this same grape makes such different wines based on terroir. Note which are fruity, which show the flavors of many different fruits at once, and which are dominated by one or two. See if you can tell why there is such a large price difference between the wines in this sample.

EXERCISE THREE: ANCIENT TO MODERN

Wines: Italian Primitivo from Puglia, Old Vine Zinfandel from Lodi, California, Old Vine Zinfandel from California, not from Lodi.

Price: Each bottle of wine should cost about $10.00 or less.

Process: Primitivo wine from Italy is one of the oldest wines. It has been consumed since the days of the Ancient Greeks. The same grape came to the United States in the past 100 years and has made a new home in California. Observe, smell, and drink the wines in the order listed. Compare and contrast the wines. The oldest expression of the wine is the Italian wine from Puglia. The winemakers in Lodi are trying their best to replicate that wine, and the Lodi climate is most like Italy's. The wine that is not from Lodi will also be trying to imitate the Italian wine but will have less similar terroir.

EXERCISE FOUR: OAK

Wines: Chablis, California Butter Chardonnay, Beaujolais, Edmundo Double Oaked Cabernet.

Price: Expect to pay $25 for the Chablis, $15 for the California Chardonnay, $20 for the Beaujolais, and $15 for the Cabernet.

Process: Compare the color of the Chablis to the California Chardonnay. Note how the oak darkens the white wine. Then smell and taste the wines to note the differences. Next, compare the lighter, fresher Beaujolais, which is a young, fresh unoaked wine, to the Cabernet. Note the difference in colors, smells, and tastes. Consider when you would prefer one of these wines versus the others. Which are better alone, which would be better with food, and what foods, and why?

Glossary of Common Wine Terms

Acidification

Acidification is a winemaking process of adding acid to a wine or grape must to increase its total acidity, which is crucial for balancing flavors, ensuring microbial stability, and improving aging potential. This technique is most often used for wines made from grapes grown in warm climates, or vintages, where grapes can become overripe, lose natural acidity, and develop a high pH. The most common acid added is tartaric acid, although other acids can also be used.

Aspect

Aspect refers to the direction a vineyard slope faces, a critical element of terroir that influences sunlight exposure, temperature, and, thus, grape ripeness. For example, in the Northern Hemisphere, south-facing slopes are preferred in cooler climates to maximize the sun's warmth and extend the growing season, while northern-facing slopes in warmer regions may be used to reduce excessive heat.

Carbonic Maceration

Whole, unbroken grape clusters are placed in a sealed, oxygen-free tank filled with carbon dioxide. Instead of yeast, enzymes within the grapes break down the sugars into alcohol, resulting in a lighter, more fruit-forward red wine with softened tannins. This process produces distinctive flavors like banana, bubblegum, and candied fruit, and the resulting wine is often best served slightly chilled. Frequently done with the gamay grape in the Beaujolais region of France.

Chaptalization

Chaptalization is the process of adding pure, dry sugar or concentrated juice to grape or fruit must to increase the potential alcohol content of the final wine, especially in cool vintages or regions where grapes don't ripen fully. The process, named after the French chemist Jean-Antoine Chaptal, aims to produce a more stable and flavorful wine by reaching a desired alcohol level that yeast can ferment from the available sugars. This technique increases the Brix (sugar content) of the juice, which, in turn, boosts the alcohol by volume (ABV) in the finished wine. This is a frequent practice when making Riesling wine in colder climates.

Decanting

Decanting wine involves transferring it from the bottle to a separate glass vessel, called a decanter, to either remove sediment from older wines or aerate younger wines to mellow tannins and release aromatics. For older, sediment-rich wines, decant slowly to separate the wine from the harmless solids. For younger, bold red wines, decant to increase air contact, which helps soften tannins and develop complex flavor.

Fortified Wine

A fortified wine is a wine to which a distilled spirit, most often brandy (which is distilled wine), has been added to increase its alcohol content and preserve it. The addition of the spirit, which is done either during or after fermentation, also affects the wine's flavor profile and often results in a higher residual sugar content. Fortified wines have both a high level of sweetness and a high alcohol by volume. Examples of fortified wines include Port, Sherry, Madeira, and Vermouth.

Malolactic Conversion

Malolactic conversion (or fermentation, MLC/MLF) is a process in winemaking where bacteria convert sharp malic acid into softer lactic acid, resulting in a rounder, smoother wine. This microbial process, carried out by Oenococcus oeni bacteria, also produces diacetyl, which adds buttery flavors to the wine. While nearly all red wines undergo MLF for greater stability and a supple texture, it is a stylistic choice for white wines; it's avoided in crisp styles like Sauvignon Blanc but encouraged in some Chardonnay wines to produce a fuller-bodied, buttery profile.

New World Wines

Wines made in places where wine was not made before 1492. These wines often feature bolder, riper fruit flavors, higher alcohol content, and fuller body compared to Old World wines, reflecting warmer climates and more experimental, less regulated winemaking practices. They are often named by the grape varietal from which they are made rather than being named after the geographic location where they were made.

Noble Rot (Botrytis)

Noble Rot is the beneficial form of a fungus called Botrytis cinerea that affects grapes. Infestation by Botrytis requires warm and humid conditions, typically around 70 degrees Fahrenheit and above 80% humidity. Grapes picked at a certain point during infestation can produce particularly fine and concentrated sweet wine. Wines produced by this method are known as "botrytized wines" and are considered a distinct category of dessert wine.

World Wines

Wines made in places where wine has been made since before 1492. They are characterized by centuries of winemaking history, a strong emphasis on terroir (soil, climate, and landscape), stricter regulations, and a focus on complexity, subtlety, minerality, and balance. These wines often have lighter bodies, higher acidity, and are often named for their region of origin, such as Bordeaux or Chianti, rather than their grape variety.

Phylloxera

Phylloxera is an insect, native to North America, which destroys grape crops. Wines native to the Americas are largely immune to it, and wines native to the Old World are not. In the mid-1800s, phylloxera destroyed almost all wine-producing grapes in France. This is called "Great French Wine Blight." It was during this time that drinking Absinthe became popular in France due to the lack of wine. During this time, phylloxera led to the devastation of the majority of European vineyards. The problem was addressed by bringing root stock from American grapes to Europe and grafting the European grapes onto the phylloxera-resistant American root stock. This is how grapes are grown today.

Primary Aroma

Primary aromas in wine, also known as varietal aromas, are the fresh, fruity, floral, or vegetal scents that come directly from the grape itself and are present when the wine is young. These aromas are inherent to the grape variety, like the blackcurrant notes in a Cabernet Sauvignon or citrus in a Riesling, and can be identified by their characteristic scent, often perceived as fresh fruit, flowers, or even herbs.

Secondary Aroma

Secondary aromas in wine are those that come from winemaking processes like fermentation and aging, rather than the grape itself. These aromas can include notes of bread, yeast, butter, and cream from fermentation and malolactic conversion, and vanilla, spice, toast, and smoke from oak aging. They represent the winemaker's influence on the wine's flavor profile.

Solara System

The Solara System is a continual aging system using many different barrels and is used in the production of all sherry. Barrels in a Solera

System are arranged in different groups. Each group contains wine of the same age. The oldest group holds the wine ready to be bottled. The barrel is never totally emptied. When a fraction of the wine is extracted from the oldest barrel for bottling, that barrel is topped off with wine from the next oldest barrel, which is younger and typically less complex. That barrel, in turn, will be filled up with wine from the barrel that is younger than it, and so on. The last criadera, which holds the youngest wine, is then topped up with the wine from the latest harvest. The process is never-ending.

Sparkling Wine

Sparkling wine is a wine with significant levels of carbon dioxide in it, making it fizzy. There are different methods used to make sparkling wine, including the Traditional/Champagne Method, the Tank Method, the Asti method, the Natural Method, and the injection method. Famous sparkling wines include Champagne, Cava, and Prosecco.

Terroir

Terroir is a French term meaning "a sense of place." It refers to the combination of natural and human factors that influence the characteristics of a wine. These factors include the soil, climate, and topography of a region, as well as traditions, viticulture, and winemaking techniques that form a wine. The concept posits that these unique site-specific conditions impart distinct flavors and aromas to the grapes, making products from that location unique and impossible to reproduce elsewhere. Each wine is an expression of a unique time and place.

Tertiary Aroma

Tertiary aromas in wine are complex fragrances that develop from the aging process of the wine, either in oak barrels or in the bottle after fermentation. These aromas, such as mushroom, leather, tobacco, vanilla, or nuts, emerge as chemical changes occur over time, transforming the wine from its initial fruity and floral primary aromas.

Whole Cluster Fermentation

Whole cluster fermentation is a winemaking technique where whole grape bunches, including their stems, are fermented together instead of being de-stemmed first. This process impacts the wine›s flavor, texture, and complexity, often adding spicy, floral, or savory notes, as well as more structured tannins. The difference between simple Whole Cluster Fermentation and carbonic maceration is that in carbonic maceration, the whole cluster fermentation is done in an air-tight environment.

How to Buy Cigars at the Grocery Store

HOW ARE CIGARS MADE?

It is thought that rolling tobacco into cigars is the oldest method of smoking tobacco and was first developed by Native Americans long before their contact with Christopher Columbus in 1492.

Today, cigars are still made by rolling leaves of tobacco together in a specific way. Cigar making does not involve chemical additives, papers, or filters; it is all-natural tobacco. The outer part of the cigar is made from a tobacco leaf called the wrapper. The wrapper contributes heavily to a cigar's appearance and flavor. A good wrapper is not full of veins and can range in color from light tan to almost black. Under the wrapper is a layer of tobacco called the binder. Binder tobacco leaves are rolled under the wrapper and influence the flavor and strength of the cigar. Inside the cigar is tobacco, called filler. This tobacco is a blend determined by the cigar maker, which determines the unique properties of that cigar. Together, the wrapper, binder, and filler combine to determine the cigar's strength, flavor profile, and nicotine level. How the cigar is made, specifically its size and shape, will determine how quickly the cigar is smoked. A quality cigar uses high-quality tobacco and is constructed well. They can come in many different lengths, widths, and shapes.

WHAT IS THE DIFFERENCE BETWEEN A CHEAP CIGAR AND AN EXPENSIVE CIGAR OTHER THAN THE PRICE?

Generally speaking, a quality cigar is hand-rolled, and a low-quality cigar is machine-made. High-quality cigars use long filler tobacco, and lower-quality cigars use short filler tobacco. You want to buy hand-rolled cigars that use long filler tobacco.

AREN'T CUBAN CIGARS THE BEST?

There is no doubt that when the average person thinks of cigars, they think of Cuba. It is true that many wonderful cigars come from that island nation, but you won't be buying them at a grocery store in the United States! The good news is that it doesn't mean you can't buy an excellent, world-class cigar at the grocery store today. The truth is that the world has never produced more high-quality cigars than it does today. The cigar industry has developed premier cigar making in places such as the Dominican Republic, Nicaragua, and Honduras so well that cigars from those places now rival the famous Cuban sticks that have made that island famous.

IF NOT CUBA, WHERE ARE THE GOOD CIGARS FROM?

You are very likely to find high-quality, hand-rolled cigars for sale at your grocery store that are from Nicaragua and from the Dominican Republic. Generally speaking, cigars from the Dominican Republic tend to be more on the mild side than cigars from Nicaragua.

The Arturo Fuente company has made the Dominican Republic famous for producing some of the world's best cigars, specifically their famous Opus X line. You are unlikely to find an Opus X at a grocery store, and its prices are so high that most people who aren't seriously into cigars wouldn't choose to shop at that price point anyway, but you can find excellent Arturo Fuente offerings in most places that sell cigars. You won't go wrong with any cigar from that company, and they offer many styles of cigar, including their Hemingway line, their 858 line, and their Grand Reserva line. If you buy a box of Fuentes for your poker game, bachelor party, or football game, no cigar-loving friend who attends will be disappointed at the quality of the offering. Other high-quality brands likely to be found in grocery stores include Ashton and Montecristo.

Cigars must be stored correctly, which means controlling humidity and temperature. Ideally, cigars will be kept in a place with humidity between 68% and 72%, with a corresponding temperature of around 65-70°F. One way to help preserve humidity levels is to store cigars in a small tube. If you see cigars for sale in their own small tube in a grocery store, this can be a sign that the cigar has been stored well.

Cigars come in many different shapes and sizes. Generally, longer and thicker cigars take longer to smoke. For most occasions, a cigar that is about 5 inches long and has a diameter a little smaller than a quarter will be a good hour-long smoke.

Cigars must be cut before being smoked. The end of the cigar that will go in the smoker's mouth is sealed by a piece of tobacco called the cap. There are many ways to cut a cigar; they include using a punch to make a small hole in the cap, using a straight cutter that looks like a small guillotine to slice the back end off cleanly, and using a V-cutter that cuts out a uniform V-shaped wedge from the back of the cigar. I suggest buying an inexpensive V-cutter. These may be had for $10 to $15 and last for years. There is no need to buy an expensive one. The V-cutter has a preformed shape and, unlike the other methods, is very easy to use without making a mistake. The cutter has an indentation in which to place the butt of the cigar. Then simply slide the blade of the cutter shut, and the V-shape wedge will be cut perfectly every time. Using a V-cutter ensures that the opening is made well and is neither too deep nor too shallow. Other cutting methods take more skill to get right. A special cigar torch is not needed to light a cigar. People have been lighting cigars with matches for hundreds of years, and that method still works fine today. If you intend to store the cigars for more than a day after you buy them, consider making a "poor man's humidor." Simply get a Ziplock bag and a Boveda pack. Boveda packs can be purchased online at retailers such as Amazon.com for about $15. You simply place this small pack in the Ziplock bag with your cigars, and the cigars will be kept at the correct humidity level.

The reader is encouraged to read cigar books written by Armando Ortiz, the owner and proprietor of Crescent City Cigars in New Orleans, Louisiana.

His shop is located in the heart of the French Quarter at 730 Orleans Street. If you are in New Orleans and need a cigar, please stop in and patronize his business. You might even meet the author of this book, enjoying a cigar at the shop with his friends!

APPENDIX TO USE WHILE BUYING WINE IN THE GROCERY STORE

℘

Traditional Wine and Food Pairing Chart

FOOD	WINE	WHY
Steak	Cabernet Sauvignon, Malbec	High Tannin wine vs. fat and protein
Roast Chicken	Beaujolais, Pinot Noir	Soft tannins go well with lean foul
Salmon, Duck	Pinot Noir	Food and wine are of equal intensity
Stilton Cheese	Port	Salty cheese vs. sweet wine
Truffles	Barolo, Barbaresco, Pinot Noir	Earthy food and earthy wine
Pasta with Tomato	Sangiovese, Barolo	Acidity of wine cuts through acidic sauce
Pasta with white sauce	Pinot Grigio	Wine's acidity cuts through cream
Fried Chicken	Sparkling Wine	Acidity and effervescence cut through the dish's richness and fat, while the bubbles cleanse the palate between bites.
Fish	Sauv. Blanc, Chenin Blanc	Acidity of wine stands up to richness of fish, minerality can stand up to brine

Practical Chart of Wine and Food Pairing at the Grocery Store

MEAL	WINE
Spaghetti, Pizza, Ziti, Tomato Pasta	Chianti (ideally riserva or classico)
BBQ Ribs or BBQ chicken, BBQ Pork	Malbec (Ideally Mendoza), Sparkling Rose
Meatloaf, Hamburgers, Ground Beef	Malbec (Ideally Mendoza)
Grilled Chicken	Pinot Grigio or Pinot Noir if it is from Russian River Valley or Oregon

MEAL	WINE
Salmon	Sauv Blanc from New Zealand or Pinot Noir, if from Russian River Valley or Oregon
Steaks	Malbec (Ideally Mendoza)
Fettuccine Alfredo (alfredo pasta)	Pinot Grigio (Ideally Italian)
Grilled Sea Food	Sauv Blanc (New Zealand)
Mac & Cheese	Riesling (off dry or dry if possible) , Cava
Fried Chicken/anything deep fried	Cava or brut sparkling wine, if Cava is not available, Pinot Grigio
Fish	Sauv Blanc (New Zealand)
Pork Chops	Tempranillo or Pinot Grigio (Ideally Italian) or Pinot Noir
Taco	Tempranillo or Riesling
Grilled Cheese	Pinot Grigio Sauv. Blanc or Pinot Noir
BLT	Sauv. Blanc, Pinot Noir, or Pinot Grigio
Sandwich (Salami or strong meats)	Chianti (Ideally riserva or classico) or Tempranillo
Sandwich Cold Cuts	Pinot Grigio

Chart Explaining Old World Wines by Grape Varietal

Location/Name of Old-World Wine	Grape Varietal	Where the Same Grapes are Used in the Rest of the World
Bordeaux	Cabernet Sauvignon, Merlot, Cabernet Franc, Petit Verdot	USA, Australia, South Africa, Chile, Bulgaria, Romania, Spain, Italy, Lebanon
Burgundy (red)	Pinot Noir	USA, New Zealand, Australia, South Africa
Burgundy (white)	Chardonnay	Australia, New Zealand, USA, South Africa, Chile, Argentina, Spain, Italy, Bulgaria, Hungary
Northern Rhône	Syrah (shiraz)	Australia, New Zealand, USA, South Africa
Alsace	Gewurztraminer, Riesling	New Zealand, Australia, USA
Sancerre	Sauvignon Blanc	New Zealand, Chile, USA, South Africa
Champagne	Chardonnay, Pinot Noir, Pinot Meunier	USA, Australia, New Zealand, South Africa

FOOD AND WINE PAIRING REMINDERS

Remember: Food impacts wine more than wine impacts food.

ABV	Sweetness Level
12.5% or more	Dry
11% to 12.5%	Off Dry
8% to 11%	Semi Sweet
8% or less	Sweet

When Pairing Wine with Food:

A. Match Intensity

B. Consider acidity (the wine should be more acidic than the food)

C. Remember tannins. The fattier the food, the more tannins the wine should have.

D. Spicy food makes the alcohol in wine seem harsh. So, serve sweeter wines with spicy food. Determine the sweetness level by using the ABV chart above.

E. Salt in food makes a wine taste less acidic, sweeter, and less bitter than it is. So, serve wines that are dry and have high acidity with salty foods.

F. Consider pairing food and wine by place of origin.

About the Author

Carl Davis lives in New Orleans, where he loves life and drinks wine.

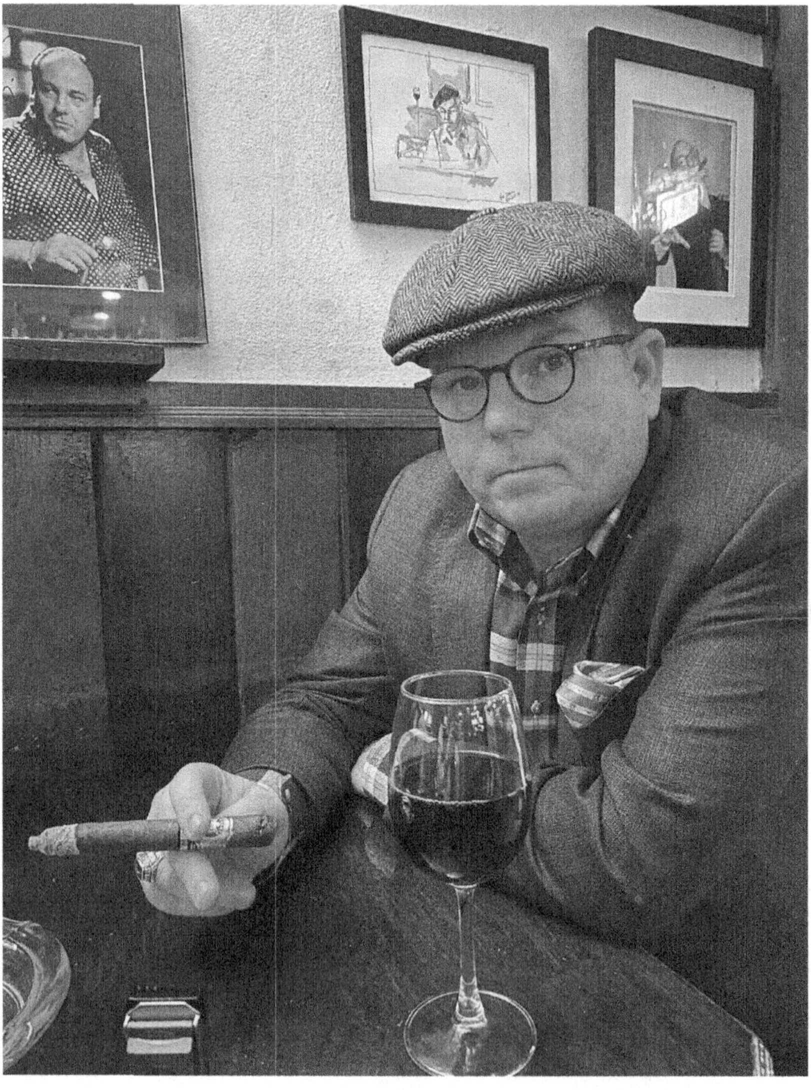

Made in the USA
Coppell, TX
19 June 2026

82418863R00069